REVERSE PAIN IN HIPS AND KNEES

Super-Effective Back, Hip, and Knee
Stretches and Strengthening Exercises

**Reverse Your Pain Series
Book 2**

Morgan Sutherland, L.M.T.

Reverse Pain in Hips and Knees

Super-Effective Back, Hip, and Knee Stretches and Strengthening Exercises

Reverse Your Pain Series Book 2

Copyright © 2019 Morgan Sutherland, L.M.T.

All rights reserved.

ISBN: 979-8-9864227-3-2

Illustrations: Copyright Morgan Sutherland

Cover image: 123RF

CONTENTS

MEDICAL DISCLAIMER

The information provided in this book is not intended to be a substitute for professional medical advice, diagnosis, or treatment. Never disregard or delay seeking professional medical advice, because of something you read in this book. Never rely on information in this book in place of seeking professional medical advice.

Morgan Sutherland is not responsible or liable for any advice, course of treatment, diagnosis, other information, services, and/or products that you obtain in this book. You are encouraged to consult with your doctor or healthcare provider with regard to the information contained in this book. After reading this book, you are encouraged to review the information carefully with your professional healthcare provider.

PERSONAL DISCLAIMER

I am not a doctor. The information I provide is based on my personal experiences and research as a licensed massage therapist. Any recommendations I make about posture, exercise, stretching, and massage should be discussed between you and your professional healthcare provider to prevent any risk to your health.

GOT BACK PAIN? NOW WHAT?

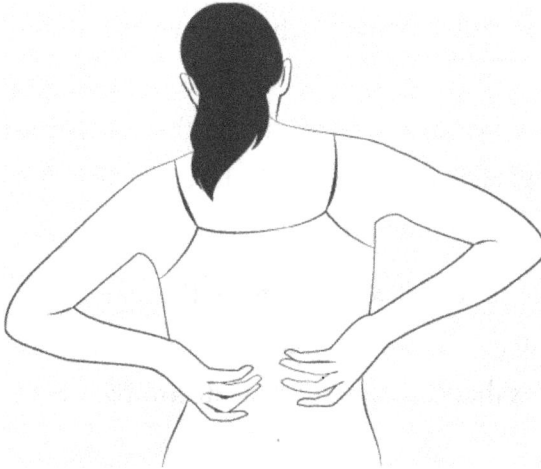

Chronic pain, affecting approximately 100 million people each year, is classified as pain persisting for 12 weeks or more. Low back pain is the most common kind of chronic pain complaint. When the body's pain signals keep firing in the nervous system for this length of time, it can have a draining effect on a person's quality of life—physically, mentally, and spiritually.

In the United States, 8 out of 10 people will experience low back pain at some time in their lives. Low back pain is the second most frequent reason for doctor visits, next to the common cold, and it is the leading cause of job-related disabilities.

When sudden and acute back pain strikes, it can cause intense shooting or stabbing pain that dramatically limits movement. This is often to the point that standing upright can feel like a Sisyphean task—repeatedly rolling the same rock up the hill without any relief. This pain can last anywhere from a few days to weeks.

Subacute back pain, pain lasting 4 to 12 weeks, is generally the result of a strained or pulled muscle—that's when the muscle or tendon is ripped or torn, from overstretching it, or by pulling the muscle in one direction while it is contracting in the other direction. Muscle strains are typically caused from a fall, careless lifting technique, poor posture, or a sudden movement.

When the muscles are strained or torn, the area around the muscles become inflamed. This inflammation leads to back spasms, and it is the back spasms that can cause both acute low back pain and difficulty moving.

Finding a quick fix for your back pain can be a slippery slope, due to all the back pain myths and misconceptions.

One truth that is certain is that regular exercise *prevents* back pain. And doctors might recommend exercise for people who have recently hurt their lower backs. The doctors will usually suggest that the person start with gentle movements and gradually build up the intensity. Once the immediate pain goes away, an exercise plan can help keep it from coming back.

The National Institute of Neurological Disorders and Stroke (NINDS) says on its website that, "*Exercise may be the most effective way to speed recovery from low back pain and help strengthen back and abdominal muscles. . . . Maintaining and building muscle strength is particularly important for persons with skeletal irregularities."*

According to health researcher Chris Maher at the University of Sydney in Australia, after analyzing 21 global studies (involving more than 30,000 participants) on how to treat and prevent lower back pain, those who use a combination of exercise and back pain education reduced the risk of repeated low back pain in the year following an episode between 25 and 40 percent. It didn't really matter what kind of exercise—core strengthening, aerobic exercise, or flexibility and stretching.

"What we do understand about the back is that the more you use it, the more likely you are to keep it strong, fit and healthy," says Maher.

See https://www.npr.org/sections/health-shots/2016/01/11/462366361/forget-the-gizmos-exercise-works-best-for-lower-back-pain

Before we get into the specific back pain exercise routine that helped fix my back pain problem, let's look at the four most common causes of back pain.

Four Most Common Causes of Back Pain

Neglected postures, such as rounding your low back while sitting for extended periods of time in front of the computer, standing for hours stooped over, sleeping improperly, and lifting poorly, can all lead to chronic back pain.

Maintaining the natural lumbar curve in your low back is essential to preventing posture-related back pain. This natural curve works as a shock absorber, helping to distribute weight along the length of your spine.

Here are the four most common causes of back pain.

#1 Postural Neglect

- Rounding your low back while sitting for extended hours in front of the computer
- Poor lifting techniques
- Prolonged forward bending while working
- Standing or lying for long periods of time in a poor position

#2 Sitting

- Slouching while sitting at a restaurant, café, or movie theater
- Sedentary office jobs that require endless hours of sitting can overstretch the back muscles, distorting the vertebrae, potentially causing bulging or herniated discs

#3 Standing (or Poor Lying Posture)

- Standing (or lying) for long periods of time, lordosis (inward curve of the spine) can become excessive and pain results
- Working in stooped positions when doing yard work or household chores, such as raking, shoveling, or vacuuming

#4 Lifting

- Lifting objects with a rounded back can put unwanted pressure on the vertebral discs. Keeping the body upright, avoiding back flexion, and maintaining a natural lordotic curve is a better option when lifting

Source: *Treat Your Own Back*

TWENTY-ONE DAY, LOW BACK PAIN, RELIEF PROGRAM

How to Use This Book

For the best results, do the exercises every day for 21 days.

All you need is a mat or comfortable surface (not a bed), such as a rug or carpet, and that's it. In addition, you need the determination and willpower to do the exercises.

Let's begin.

The Stretching Routine

For the first exercise, you're going to stretch your quadriceps muscles (thighs).

Sitting for long periods of time puts the quadriceps in a constant contraction, keeping them short and tight.

Of the four quadriceps muscles, only one of them, the rectus femoris, attaches at the hip near the knee.

Tight quadriceps pull the pelvis forward at the front part of your hips, called the anterior superior iliac spine (ASIS). This pulling tilts the pelvis downward or forward, resulting in what's called an anterior pelvic tilt.

This anterior tilt increases the arch in the lower back (referred to as lordosis), and this can make the back muscles tight and sore. Inadvertently, the tight quads can weaken or overstretch the hamstrings.

Good postural alignment, stretched-out quads, and strong hamstrings will help to balance and protect the low back muscles and keep them pain free.

1a. Couch Potato Quad Stretch (version 1)

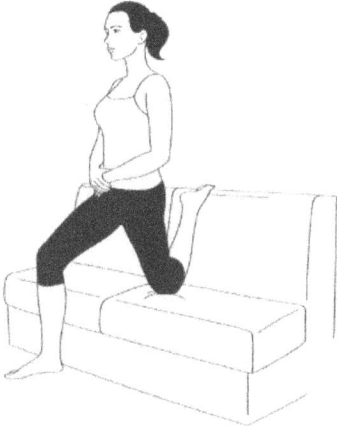 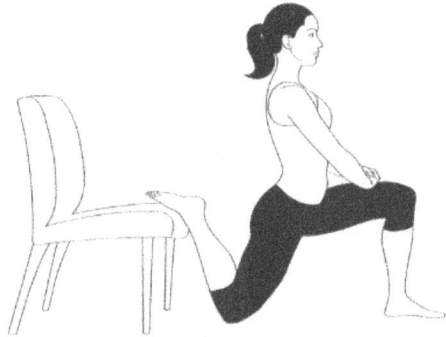

version 1   version 2

Start by placing your left knee on the couch cushion, with your left foot against the back of the couch. The closer your knee is to the back cushion, the more intense a stretch it will be; the farther from the back cushion, the easier it is.

If this is too painful for the top of your foot, place a rolled-up towel or small pillow underneath that foot/ankle.

Once you've gotten into this position, SLOWLY bring the right leg into a lunge, making sure that the knee is over the ankle and not past the toes.

From here, kick your left foot into the back cushion to contract (resist) the muscles on the front of the leg (quadriceps).

As you kick into the back cushion, use your other leg to push your body back to stretch the quads. As you go back, be sure to tuck the glutes under (the opposite of sticking your butt out) in order to increase the stretch.

Move back and forth for 1 minute.

Repeat on the other leg.

1b. Couch Potato Quad Stretch (version 2)

If no couch is available, a chair will do the trick.

See https://premiersportsandspine.com/2015/06/the-best-stretch-for-your-hip-flexors-the-couch-stretch/

2a. Hip Flexor Stretch

Did you know that a tight psoas could be causing your back pain?

The psoas muscle is a major hip flexor, located deep in the abdominal contents and spans from the upper portion of the femur to the lumbar vertebrae. It affects your posture and helps to stabilize your spine.

The psoas enables you to walk and run. Every time you lift your knee, it contracts. When your leg swings back, the psoas lengthens.

The psoas often gets short from too much sitting. If your psoas is tight and in a contracted state, it will bring your lower back forward, moving you into an anterior tilt: creating a lordotic curve. This pressure can ultimately compress the joints and discs of the lumbar vertebrae and cause degeneration, which will make them more susceptible to injury.

So regularly stretching your psoas can help prevent future injuries from occurring, or it can mend a chronically tight psoas.

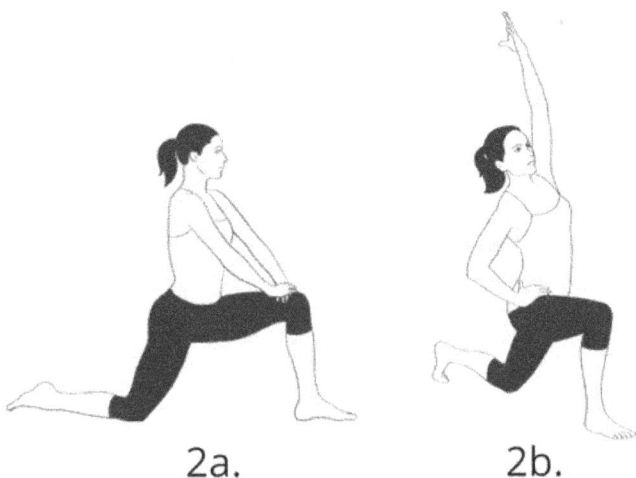

2a.   2b.

To effectively stretch the hip flexors, first kneel on your right knee, with toes down, and place your left foot flat on the floor in front of you.

Place both hands on your left thigh and press your hips forward until you feel a good stretch in the hip flexors.

Contract your abdominals and slightly tilt your pelvis back, while keeping your chin parallel to the floor. Hold this pose for 20 to 30 seconds, and then switch sides.

2b. Hip Flexor Stretch (with Arm Raised over Head)

First, kneel on your right knee, with toes down, and place your left foot flat on the floor in front of you.

Place both hands on your left thigh and press your hips forward until you feel a good stretch in the hip flexors.

Reach your hands (one or both) over your head and arch your body back.

Contract your abdominals and slightly tilt your pelvis back while keeping your chin parallel to the floor. Hold this pose for 30 seconds, and then switch sides. Stretch your nondominant side first.

Source: *The Four-Hour Body*, p. 352.

3. Adductor Stretches

The inner thigh muscles, known as the adductors, play a crucial role in movement and stabilization of the legs and pelvis. The adductors help support the pelvis and allow you to bring your legs toward and across the midline of your body.

Tight adductors can distort the posture and accentuate the anterior tilt, which contributes to low back pain.

Weak adductors can throw off a person's gait and force the body to compensate so as to maintain pelvic stability.

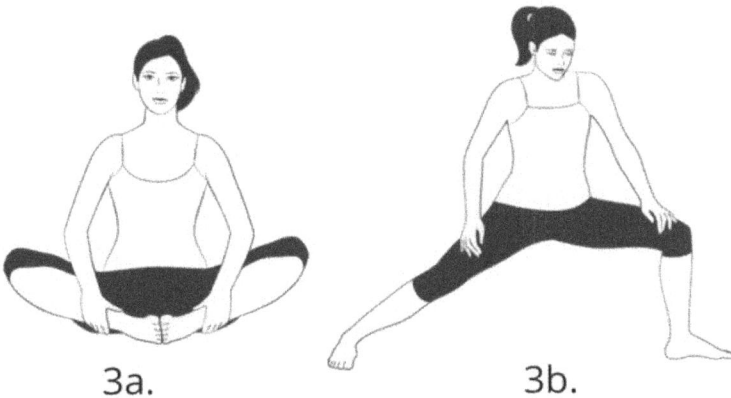

3a.   3b.

3a. Butterfly Stretch

The butterfly stretch is a static stretch that helps to improve the flexibility of your adductors.

First, sit on the floor or a mat. Open your hips, flex your knees, and move your feet together. Grasp your ankles and gently pull them up, as you simultaneously push your elbows into your knees. Hold for 30 seconds.

3b. Sideways Lunge Adductor Stretch

If you prefer to do this adductor stretch standing, then the sideways lunge is for you. Keep the rear foot sideways and flat on the floor, and gently bend the front leg until you feel a mild stretch along the inside of your leg.

Keep your body upright—there is no need to lean forward. Hold this stretch for 30 seconds.

Repeat with your other leg.

4. Hamstring Stretches

Desk jockeys who sit all day long are guaranteed to have tight hamstrings. These are the group of muscles that help bend your knee and extend your hips. They are located on the back of your upper thigh.

When the hamstrings are too tight, they can pull the backside of the pelvis downward. This downward pull of the pelvis can cause a flattening of your back, which increases pressure on the bones of your lumbar spine.

If this pulling happens for an extended time period, it causes the muscles in the low back, which hold your body upright, to become weak and start to fatigue, as they try to hold your body upright against gravity. For this reason, stretching the hamstrings is crucial to help reduce the strain on your low back.

4a. Static Hamstring Stretch (Lying Down)

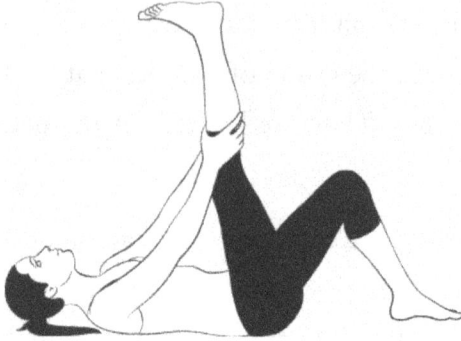

Grab the back of your leg with both hands. Pull your leg toward you gently, while keeping both hips on the floor.

Hold for 30 seconds. Contract your abdominals when bringing your legs up.

Repeat on the other leg.

4b. Hamstring Stretch with Yoga Strap (Contract-Relax)

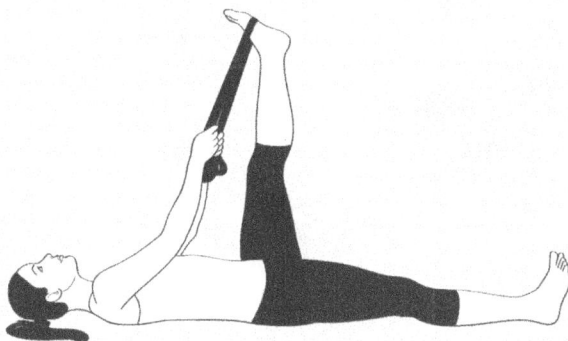

Using a yoga strap or stretch strap has been shown to be extremely effective at increasing the hamstring's flexibility and restoring range of motion.

To perform a proprioceptive neuromuscular facilitation (PNF) hamstring stretch (contract-relax antagonist-contract) using a strap, lie on your back and loop the strap around the ball of your foot, holding the ends of the strap with both hands.

Try to keep your chin down and your shoulders back. Exhale, while pushing your heel up toward the ceiling. Hold this stretch for 20 to 30 seconds.

Keeping your knee straight, push down with your heel into the strap toward the floor for 3 to 5 seconds. Then try to straighten your knee and actively push your foot toward the ceiling, contracting your quadriceps. Hold this for 3 to 5 seconds.

Relax and then hold this stretch for 20 to 30 seconds.

Repeat on the other leg.

See http://www.stretching-exercises-guide.com/hamstring-stretches.html

5. Piriformis Stretch

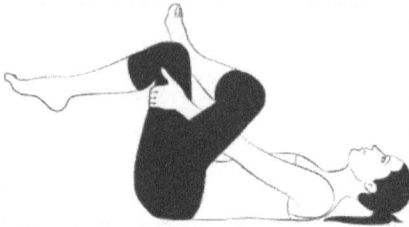
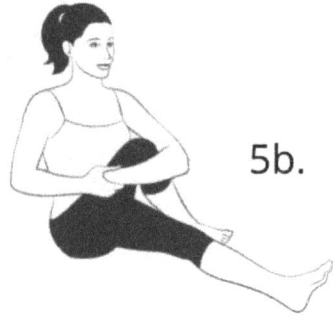

5a.

5b.

5a. Piriformis Stretch (Lying Down)

The piriformis is a tiny, pear-shaped muscle deep in the glutes that helps laterally rotate the hip. If gets too tight, it can impinge the sciatica nerve that runs through or under it, causing tremendous pain, tingling, and numbness through the glutes and into the lower leg. This condition is called piriformis syndrome. When performing the piriformis stretch, make sure to contract your abdominals before crossing your leg and resting your foot on the other knee. Hold this stretch for 30 seconds.

Repeat with your other leg.

5b. Piriformis/ Glute Stretch (Sitting)

While in a sitting position, cross your right leg over your straightened left leg. Hug your right knee with your left arm, making sure to keep your back straight.

Hold this stretch for 30 to 60 seconds.

Repeat on the opposite side.

6. Spinal Rotation and Twist

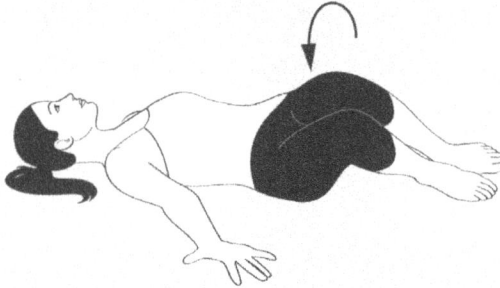

Lie on your back with your feet flat on the floor and gently drop your knees side to side. Draw in your abdominal muscles, like a vacuum, and maintain this contraction throughout the exercise.

Slowly rotate your knees to the right, making sure to keep your hips in contact with the floor. Engage your lateral abdominals (obliques) to help you pull your knees back to the center

Repeat on the opposite side.

Repeat 10 to 20 times.

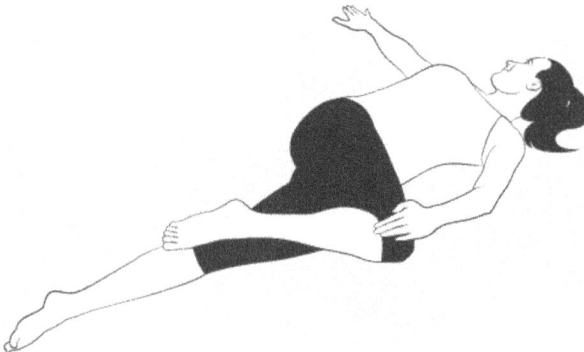

Remain on the floor and stretch both legs out. With your right arm stretched to the right, lift your right knee across your left knee.

Contract your abdominals before bringing your knee up and over the leg. Hold for 20 seconds.

Repeat this move with the other knee.

7. Cat and Cow Pose

Starting on your hands and knees, move into the Cat Pose by slowly pressing your spine up, arching your back.

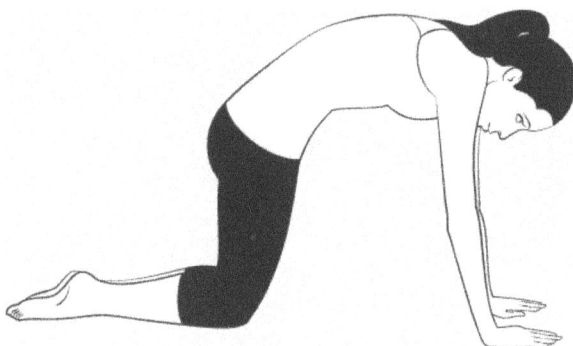

Hold the pose for a few seconds.

Then move to the Cow Pose by scooping your spine in, pressing your shoulder blades back, and lifting your head.

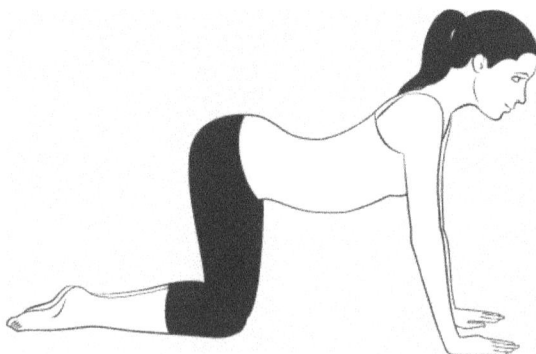

Moving back and forth from Cat Pose to Cow Pose helps move your spine to a neutral position, relaxing the muscles and easing tension.

Repeat the sequence 10 times, flowing smoothly from cat to cow, and cow back to cat.

8. Press Up

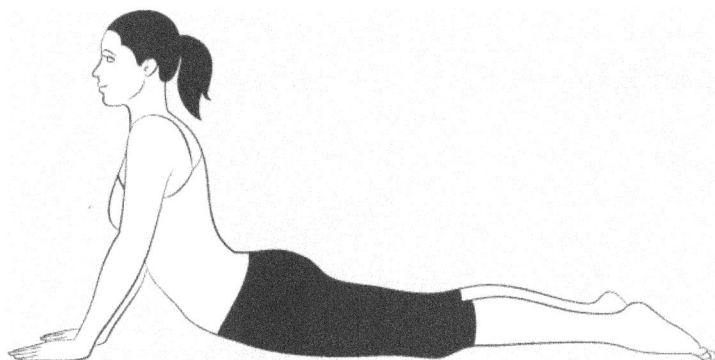

Press your palms into the floor and lift your upper body, keeping hips and pelvis rooted to the floor. Extend through the spine from the tailbone to the neck, allowing your back to arch.

Hold for 2 seconds, and then slowly lower to the start position for one rep. Do 10 reps.

9. Quadratus Lumborum (QL) Stretch

Lie on your side with your forearm on the floor under your shoulder to prop you up, and then stack your legs on top of each other.

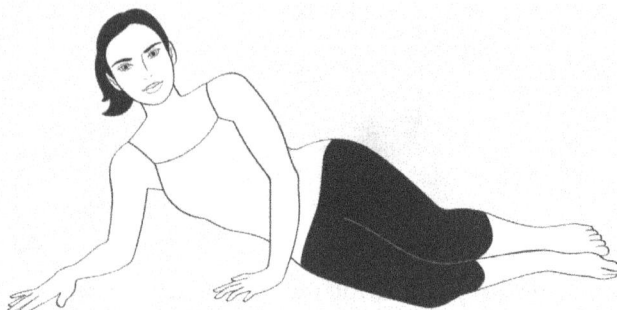

Push up as shown, keeping your hips on the floor. You'll feel the stretch in your QL.

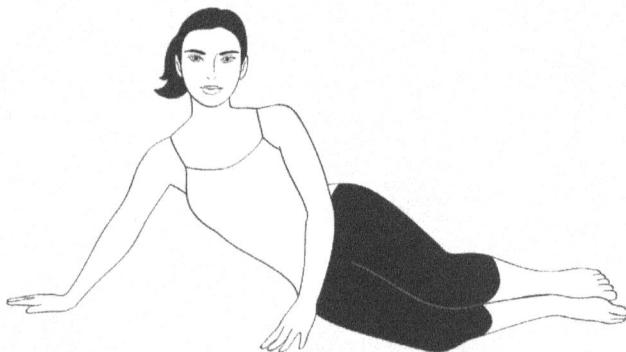

Hold the stretch for 30 seconds.

Repeat on the opposite side.

Build a Strong Core

Sedentary lifestyles usually go hand in hand with being unfit and overweight. According to a study published in the *American Journal of Epidemiology*, obese people have a higher prevalence of low back pain than non-overweight individuals do.

Another study, published in the *Arthritis & Rheumatology* journal, reported that overweight and obese adults are more likely to have disc degeneration in their low back than normal-weight adults are. An excessive anterior tilt in the pelvis, coupled with weak abdominal muscles creates an excessive amount of tension in a person's low back. This leads to back pain and the increased likelihood of disc deterioration.

So, it's no secret. If your back is sore and achy, you need to strengthen your core, the abdominal and pelvic muscles that encircle and support the spine.

The "core" consists of specific muscles, which stabilize the spine and pelvis, and run the entire length of the torso. The core muscles make it possible to stand upright, shift your body weight, transfer your energy, and move in any direction.

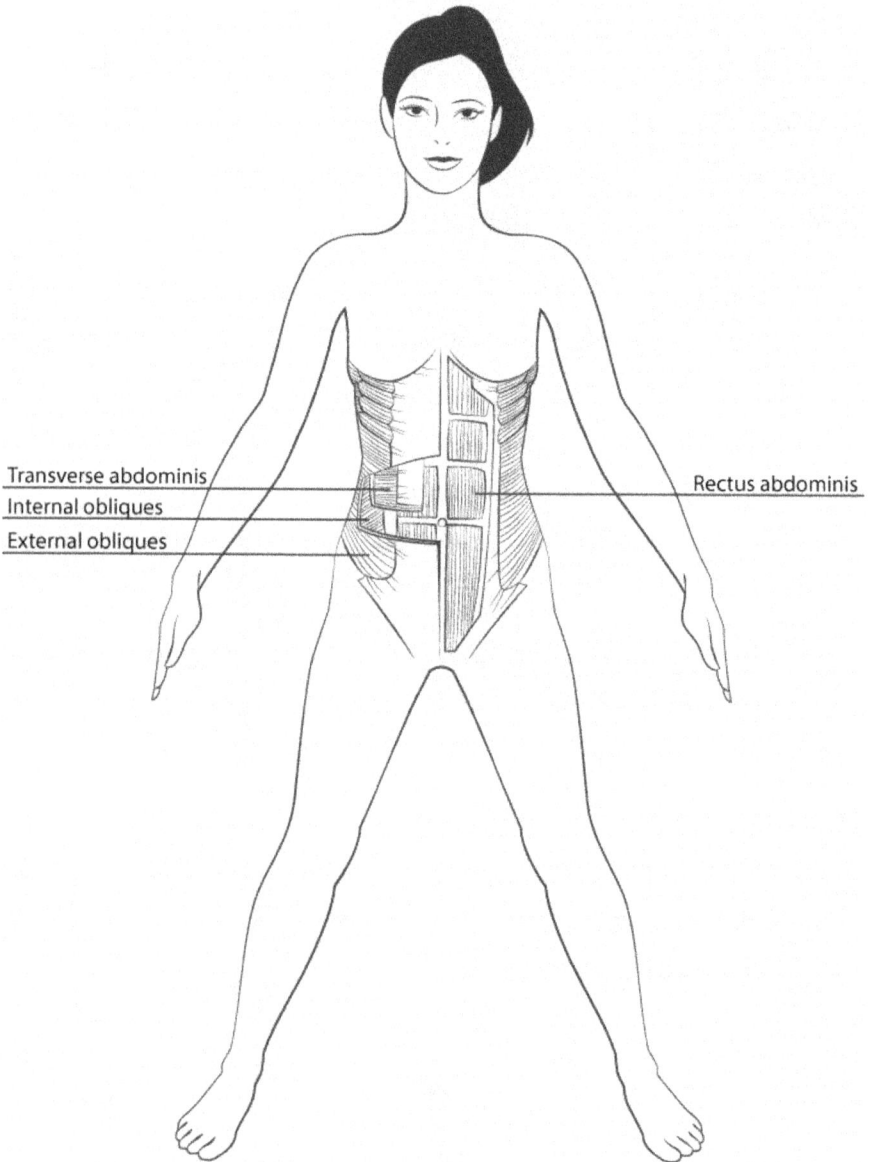

Transverse abdominis
Internal obliques
External obliques

Rectus abdominis

There are four major core muscles: the rectus abdominis, external and internal obliques, and the transverse abdominis.

The rectus abdominis extends along the front of the abdomen and forms the "six-pack" muscles.

The external obliques are on the side and front of the abdomen, around the waist.

Underneath the external obliques are the internal obliques. Underneath the internal obliques is the transverse abdominis, which wraps around your spine for protection and stability.

Muscles function with an agonist/antagonist response, so if one muscle takes the brunt of the work, the neglected muscle becomes weakened. Weak core muscles diminish a person's natural lumbar curve, creating a scenario for crippling back pain. A strong, balanced core helps maintain appropriate posture and reduces strain on the spine.

10. Pelvic Tilt Warm-Up Exercises

10a. Abdominal Draw In

Lie on your back with your knees bent and feet flat on the floor. In this relaxed position, the small of your back will not be touching the floor.

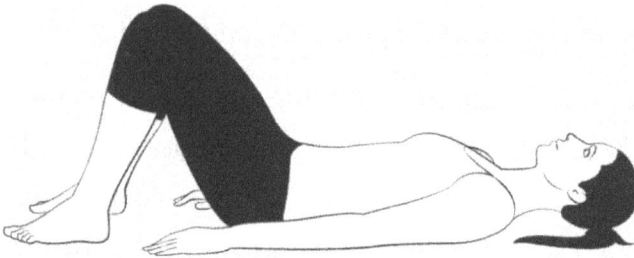

Take a deep breath and on the exhale, pull your abdominals in and push your low back toward the floor.

Repeat 20 times.

10b. Abdominal Draw In with Knee to Chest

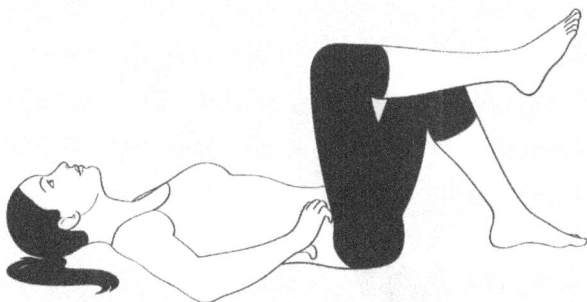

Lie on your back and draw one knee to the chest, while maintaining the abdominal draw in; do not grab the knee with your hand.

Repeat 10 to 20 times with each leg.

10c. Abdominal Draw In with Double Knee to Chest

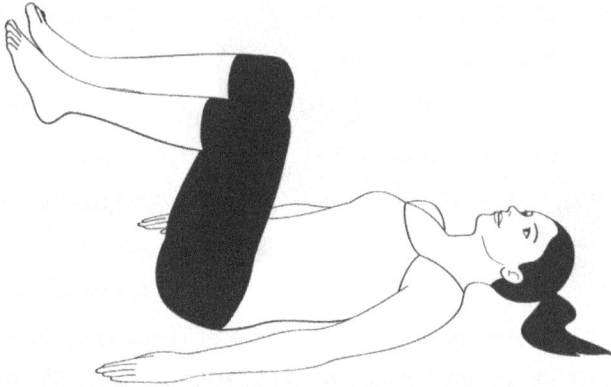

Bring both knees to your chest at the same time. Maintain the abdominal draw in throughout the entire exercise.

Repeat 10 to 20 times.

11. The Plank

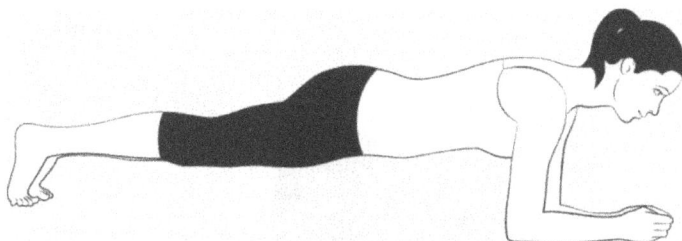

Get into a plank position on the floor with feet hip-width apart and elbows directly under your shoulders.

Brace your core by contracting your abs and attempt to bring your belly button toward your spine.

Keep your back straight and legs and glutes engaged the entire time. Hold this pose for 1 minute.

If 15 to 30 seconds is all you can do, that's fine, just stay at it. The plank exercise works the transverse abdominis and this helps you sit up straight, hold your shoulders back, and prevent forward head posture.

You might feel sore, but stay at it. In time you'll be able to work your way up to 1 minute.

12. The Side Plank

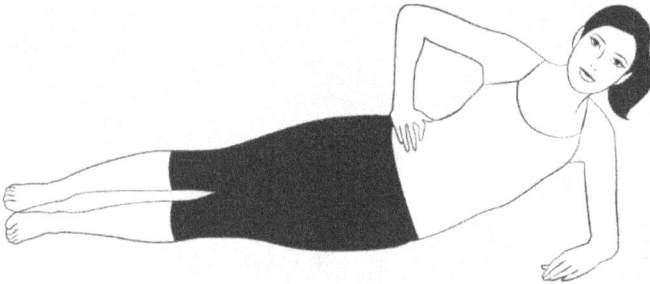

When performing the side plank, start by lying on your side with your forearm on the floor under your shoulder to prop you up, and then stack your feet on top of each other.

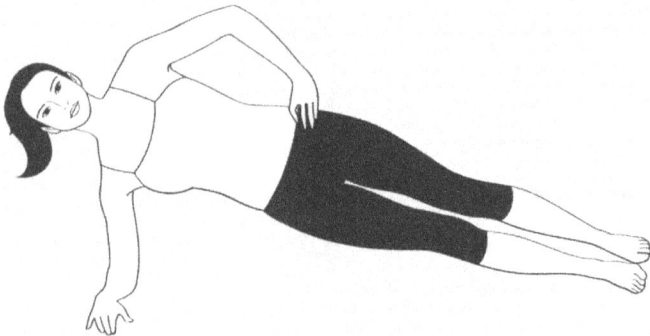

Contract your abdominals and press your forearm into the floor to raise your hips, so that your body is straight from your ankles to your shoulders.

Hold this position for 30 to 60 seconds.

Repeat on the other side.

13. Adductor Assisted Back Extension

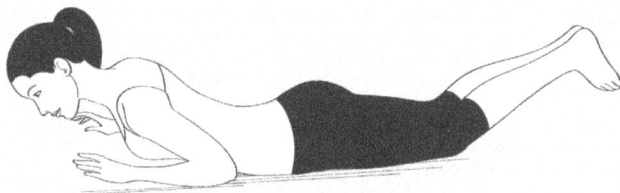

This back extension with raised and squeezed legs works the adductor muscles inside your thighs. The adductors originate in the pelvis and attach to the knee. Contracting these muscles pulls the pelvis down and alleviates compression of the lower spine.

Start by lying flat on your stomach with palms on the floor by your shoulders. Pull your elbows back against your rib cage and your arms up off the ground. Bring your feet and knees firmly together.

Then bend your knees at a 45-degree angle while pressing your knees and feet together as tightly as possible. Lower your feet until they are 6 inches off the ground. Lift your chest as high as you can, while you continue to hold your feet off the ground. Hold the pose for 10 to 15 seconds and drop down.

Repeat for another 10 to 15 seconds.

See https://www.youtube.com/watch?v=mZr5ywYLSwQ

Source: Eric Goodman, *Foundation*, pp. 96–97

14. Alternating Superman (or Superwoman) Exercise

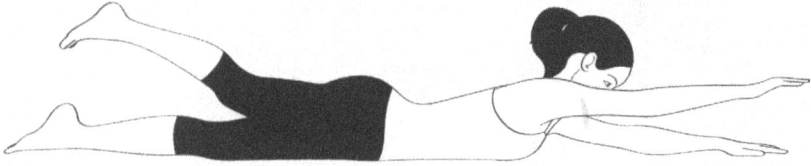

This exercise strengthens the erector spinae back muscles.

Lie face down on the floor on your stomach with arms and legs extended and your neck in a neutral position.

Lift opposite arm and leg for 3 to 5 seconds.

Repeat 10 to 20 times.

Repeat with the opposite arm and leg.

15. Bird Dog (Kneeling Superman)

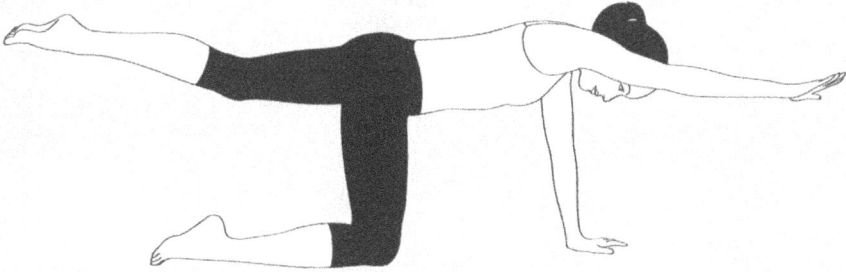

Start with the all-fours position, tighten your hamstrings, glutes, and low back. Lift to straighten your leg and opposite arm, while maintaining proper alignment. Make sure to push through your heel.

Hold for 5 seconds.

Repeat 6 to 10 times per side.

If you need to modify this exercise, you can focus on extending your legs, one at a time, and not extend your arms.

16. Active Bridge with Knee Pillow Squeeze

One of the major causes of low back pain is a weak posterior chain (glutes and hamstrings). The muscles in the front of the body—like the hip flexors and the quadriceps (the anterior kinetic chain)—tend to be stronger, tighter, and shorter than muscles in the back of the body. Sedentary lifestyle, coupled with poor sitting posture, can cause these muscle imbalances.

Bridge exercises reduce back pain by strengthening the glutes and hamstrings and evening out this muscle imbalance.

See http://backpainsolutionsonline.com/announcements-and-releases/backpain/lower-back-pain-causes/weak-posterior-kinetic-chain-cause-of-lower-back-pain

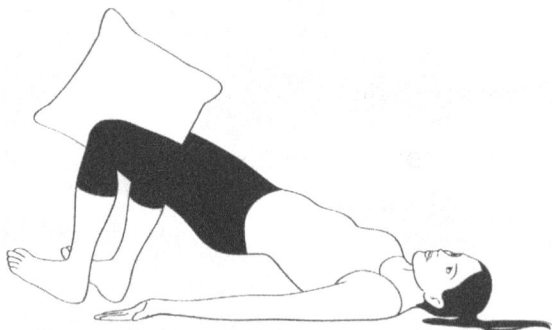

Lie on your back with your knees bent to 90 degrees, aligned with your hips, with a pillow or ball squeezed between your knees.

Press heels into the ground and lift your hips as high as you can, and then slowly lower them. Try to make this a smooth, continuous movement.

Repeat 15 times.

Do three sets.

17. Bridge with Single Leg Butt Lift

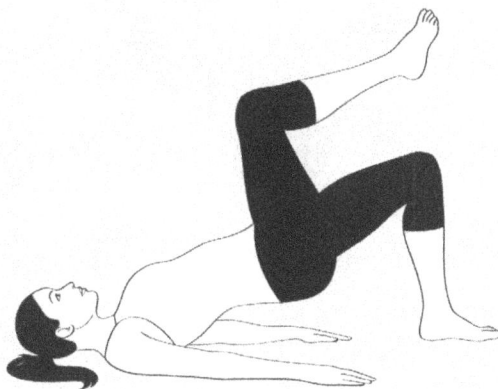

Slowly raise your butt off the floor by using your glutes and hamstrings until your torso is in line with your thighs. Hold for 3 to 5 seconds.

Repeat 10 to 20 times on each leg.

Finish with Knees to Chest Stretch

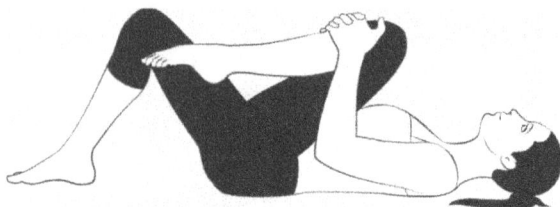

While you're still on your back, with your knees bent, grasp your left knee and pull it to your chest.

Hold for 20 seconds.

With your abdominals contracted, try to straighten your right leg. If you experience any discomfort in your back, leave your right leg bent.

Repeat this move with the other leg.

SIX FOAM ROLLING MOVES TO CONQUER BACK PAIN

Myofascial foam rolling can help break down adhesions and scar tissue in the soft tissues of the muscles. Using the weight of your own body, a cylindrical foam roller (purchase this at a fitness center, athletic store, department store, or online) can provide a myofascial release self-massage, smoothing the trigger points, while increasing blood flow and circulation to the soft tissues.

Researchers at Memorial University in Canada published a paper in the January 2014 edition of *Medicine & Science in Sports & Exercise* on the effects of foam rolling as a recovery tool after intense physical activity. The researchers found that foam rolling was beneficial at improving range of motion and reducing delayed onset muscle soreness felt immediately after a hard workout.

When using a foam roller, search for tender areas or trigger points and roll onto these areas, controlling the intensity with your own body weight. Depending on the muscle that you're targeting, you might have to position the roller in a parallel or perpendicular direction, or at a 45-degree angle.

When you find a tender spot, hold sustained pressure on it for a minimum of 20 to 90 seconds until it "releases." For this to be effective, an individual must be able to relax and breathe while the roller is on a tender spot.

When Is the Best Time to Foam Roll?

After a workout. "Foam rolling 'turns on' your parasympathetic nervous system which is responsible for helping you unwind and recover," says Dr. Kelly Starrett, physical therapist and author of *Becoming a Supple Leopard.*

1. Low Back

With the foam roller resting underneath your low back, pull your right leg up and hug your right knee for 20 seconds. Then roll from the base of your left side of your rib cage to above your glutes.

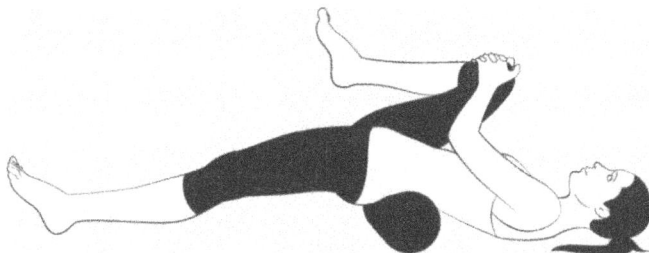

Do 10 to 12 slow and steady passes.

Repeat on the other side.

2. Glutes

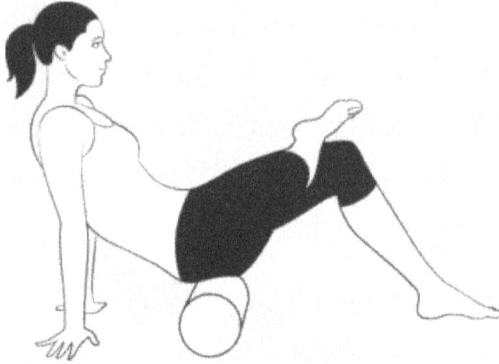

With the foam roller resting underneath both your glutes, bring your right leg up and rest your right ankle above your left knee. Roll onto the side of your right hip.

Do 10 to 12 slow and steady passes.

Repeat on the other side.

3. Hamstrings

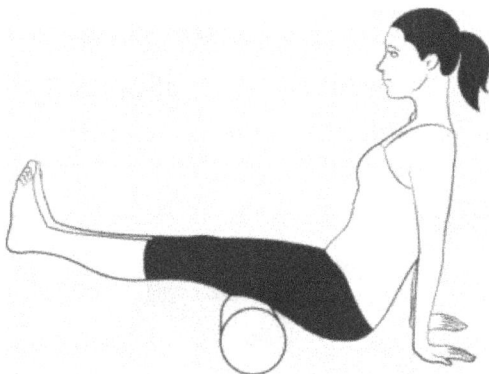

Place the foam roller underneath your upper muscles below your glutes. Cross your right leg over your left leg and roll the foam roller from your glutes down to right above your left knee.

Do 10 to 12 slow and steady passes.

Repeat on the other side.

See https://www.youtube.com/watch?v=fMfe6DnlGvA

4. Quadriceps and Hip Flexors

Because your hip flexors are located slightly toward the outer portion of your pelvic region, it's more effective to roll with just one thigh rather than on both sides at the same time.

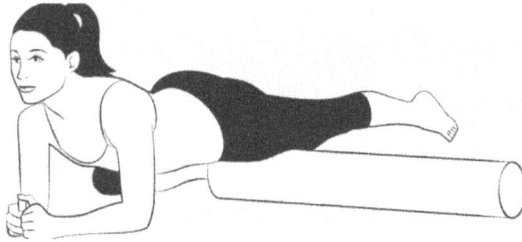

Start face down on the floor in a plank position with one thigh on the foam roller. As you roll up and down on your hip flexors, slightly rotate right to left to seek and destroy any knots or trigger points. Continue until you hit the entire front side of your thigh.

Do 10 to 12 slow and steady passes up and down the quad.

Repeat on the other side.

5. Foam Roll along Length of Back

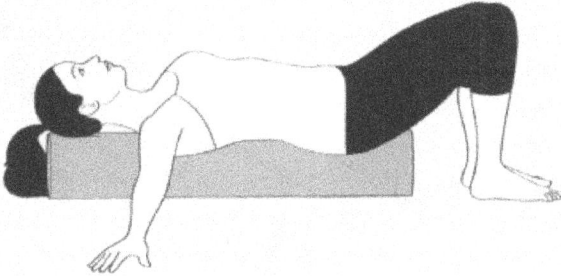

Place the foam roller vertically. Lay down on it with your head at one end and backside at the other end.

Let your arms relax to side with your palms up or down.

Lie there for up to 15 minutes.

6. Foam Roll Spinal Release

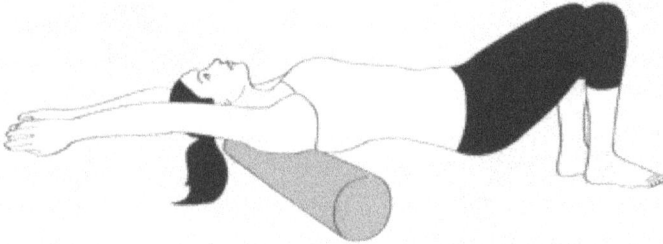

With this foam roller stretch, you won't be rolling at all; you'll be using your arms for the movement. Place your arms down at your sides. Keeping them completely straight, lift them up and over your head until they are touching the floor behind you (like you're raising your arms in excitement). You can also raise them sideways, mimicking a snow angel type of movement.

Helpful Tip: Make sure you relax your body and completely open your chest, so that you're making the most out of this exercise. The key here is to stretch and relax your muscles; you're not massaging anything with this exercise.

If you find the foam roller too big to roll out the knots in your mid and lower back, try using the time-tested tennis ball method.

Stretching is not enough when it comes to releasing a knotted muscle. If you can't carve out the time to schedule a professional, deep-tissue massage, or you can't fit one into your budget, performing a self-massage with a tennis ball or foam roller can be a cost-effective alternative.

WHAT CAN JELLY DONUTS TEACH YOU ABOUT BULGING AND HERNIATED DISCS?

Using the analogy of the jelly donut is an easy way to visualize the more complex anatomy of spinal discs. Simply put, the spinal discs are made up of two main parts—the jelly-like disc center, called the nucleus pulposus, and the outermost layer of collagen rings, called the annulus fibrosis. These two parts help the discs move and protect the vertebrae.

WHAT CAUSES A DISC TO HERNIATE OR "GO OUT" AND HOW TO FIX IT

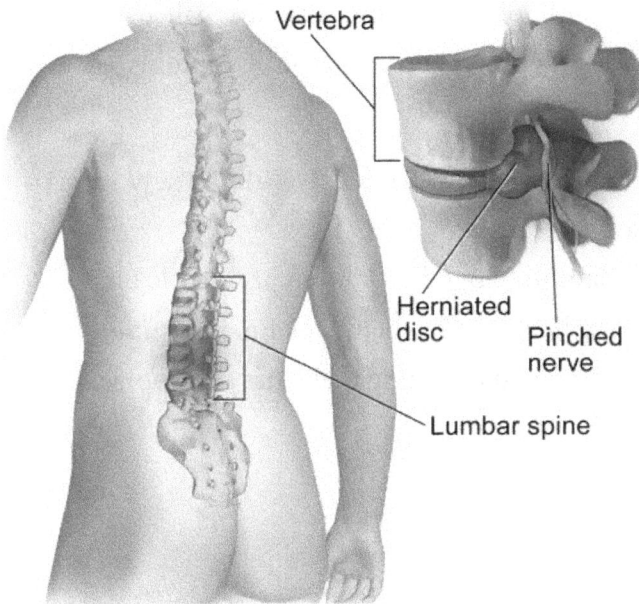

When someone has a **bulging disc**, the outer layer of the spinal disc extends outside the vertebral space, resembling a hamburger that's too big for its bun (that's right, another fast-food analogy). Research indicates that more than 50 out of 100 people who had a pain-free back and had a magnetic resonance imaging (MRI) tested positive for a bulging disk. A bulging disc is considered to be a common part of the disc's aging process and usually doesn't cause any pain.

A **slipped or herniated disc** is a whole other ball game. This happens when the tough outer layer of the disc degenerates, or sustains a trauma and cracks, allowing some of the nucleus pulposa to protrude out of the disc into the spinal canal. Herniations are most common in the fourth and fifth lumbar vertebrae. This weak spot lies directly under the spinal nerve root, putting direct pressure on the nerves causing radiating pain, tingling, and numbness down the leg.

These symptoms of a herniated disc are called sciatica or lumber radiculopathy. Some other common symptoms of a disc tear or herniated disc are . . .

- The pain came on suddenly without any injury or physical trauma.
- It's painful to bend over, even just a little bit.
- Sitting hurts, even when done for a few minutes.
- Sneezing and coughing make the pain worse.

The Six-Minute Emergency Back Pain Treatment That's Safe for Herniated and Bulging Discs

The following two exercises can push a herniated lumber disc back into place.

When your back is in an acute phase with a painful back spasm, and it hurts to even tie your shoes, before you do any stretching or strengthening exercises, you want to first decrease the level of pain.

The following exercises are taken from *Treat Your Own Back* by Robin McKenzie, a New Zealand-born physiotherapist whose McKenzie Method is currently the most studied diagnostic treatment system for back pain.

Repeat these two exercises 6 to 8 times throughout the day until you go to bed.

1. Press Up on Elbows

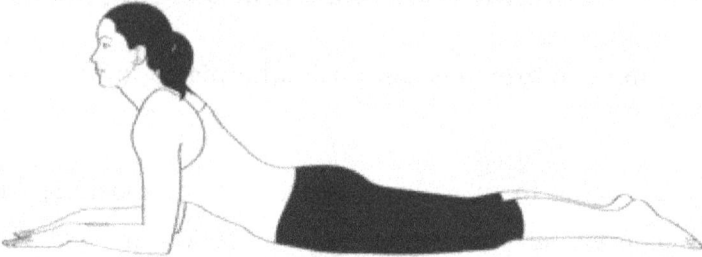

Lie on your stomach on the floor with legs extended and hands palm down just above shoulders. Retract your shoulder blades down and in toward the midline of your spine. Maintaining that position, lift your chest off the floor and extend through the spine from your tailbone to the top of your neck; allow your back to arch.

Remain in this position for 2 to 3 minutes, keeping the back of your neck long and making sure your front hip bones stay in contact with the floor during the entire movement.

2. Fully Extended Press Up

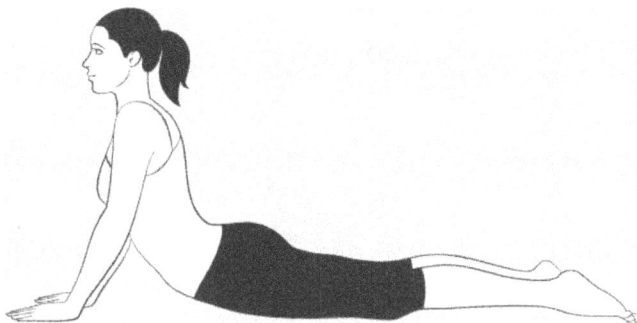

Press your palms into the floor and lift your upper body, keeping hips and pelvis rooted to the floor. Extend through the spine from the tailbone to the neck, allowing your back to arch.

Hold for 2 seconds, and then slowly lower to the start position for one rep.

Do 10 reps.

How do you know it's working?

You know it's improving when the pain moves out of the leg and/or hip region and into the center of the low back. Or if the pain's already in the center of your back, it becomes more focused into a small point. This is what Robin McKenzie refers to as "centralization."

If you get the pain to centralize, you're effectively pushing the protruding jelly back inside the spinal disc and safely away from the nearby nerves.

If at any point while you're doing the press-up exercise, you feel radiating pain down your leg, then stop.

In this case, you should lie face down on your stomach for 5 to 10 minutes, and then slowly make an effort to do the press up on elbows and then gradually move into the fully extended press up.

If the pain persists to shoot down the leg, or the sciatic leg pain worsens, contact your doctor.

GOT SCIATICA OR SI JOINT PAIN?

Sciatica is more than just a simple pain in the butt. When it strikes, it causes misery and debilitating pain that instantly downgrades your life.

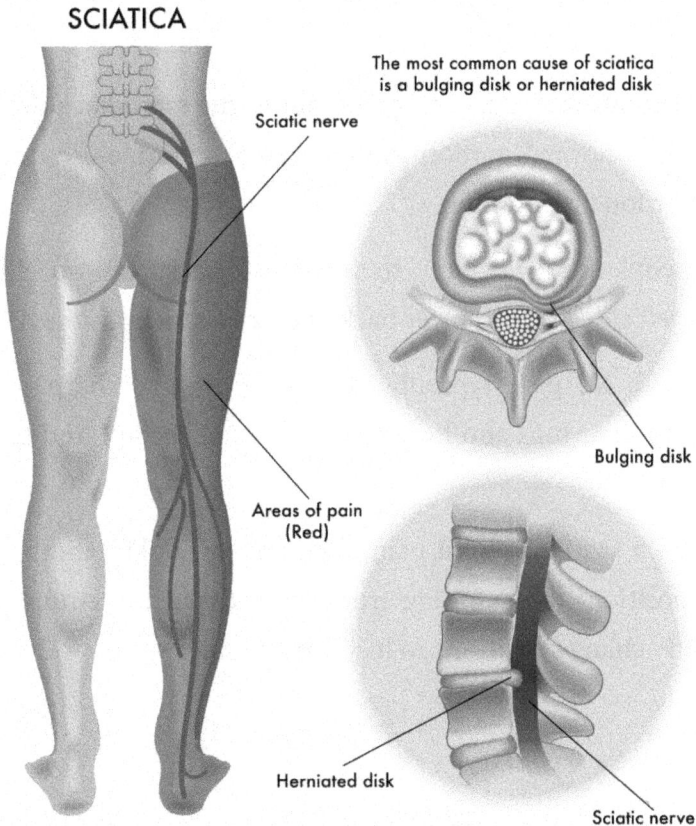

SCIATICA

Sciatic nerve

The most common cause of sciatica is a bulging disk or herniated disk

Bulging disk

Areas of pain (Red)

Herniated disk

Sciatic nerve

The sciatic nerve runs right through this tiny, but powerful muscle in your buttocks called the piriformis. The piriformis is a tiny, pear-shaped muscle deep in the glutes that helps laterally rotate the hip.

If it gets too tight, it can impinge the sciatica nerve that runs through or under it, causing shooting "electric" pain, tingling and numbness through the glutes and into the lower leg and even lead to leg weakness.

According to Spine-health.com, sciatica is most commonly caused by a herniated disc in the lumbar spine, as well as lumbar degenerative disc disease, spondylolisthesis, spinal stenosis, or osteophytes and arthritis in the spine.

Sacroiliac joint (SIJ) pain refers to pain in the sacroiliac joint region caused by abnormal motion in the sacroiliac joint, either too much motion or too little motion.

When people have SIJ pain, they feel low back pain on either the right or left side of their lower back and occasionally in the middle.

People with SIJ pain typically experience dull or sharp pain that radiates to their hips and lower back, front of the leg, and even into their groin.

People with sacroiliac joint pain often have trouble standing from a sitting position, transitioning from lying down to getting up, and frequently change positions to feel comfortable.

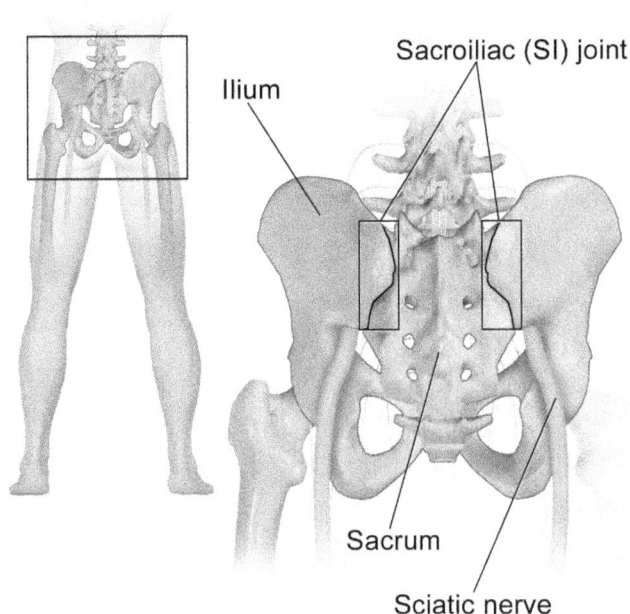

The sacroiliac joint can be found at the bottom of the spine and connects the sacrum to the pelvic bone, also known as the iliac crest, on the right and left sides at the sacroiliac joints.

These joints act as shock-absorbing structures, providing cushion between the bones, which allows the hips to move.

Some things that can irritate the sacroiliac joint and result in low back pain would include the wear and tear of aging, injury of the joint due to a fall or severe impact, an abnormal gait (how a person walks), certain medical conditions, or loosening ligaments due to hormone changes during pregnancy.

Women are 8 to 10 times more likely to have sacroiliac joint pain than men are, due to the structural and hormonal differences between the sexes.

Often confused with sciatica, SIJ pain doesn't usually travel lower than the knee. True sciatic pain symptoms commonly radiate below the knee all the way to the foot.

Another distinguishing feature of SIJ pain is that the pain is more noticeable or tender on one side over the region of the posterior superior iliac spine (PSIS), the large bumps or dimples on either side of the lower back.

This one-sided low back pain almost always presents on the same side as the "pseudo sciatica." If the muscles around this area are tight and sore, it's an indication that the SIJ is not functioning correctly.

SI JOINT SELF-ADJUSTMENT

Before we get into the reverse sciatica exercise routine, you'll want to fix your pelvic rotation with two simple self-adjustment techniques.

If you're feeling pain on the left lower side of your back, then here's what you do.

Technique #1

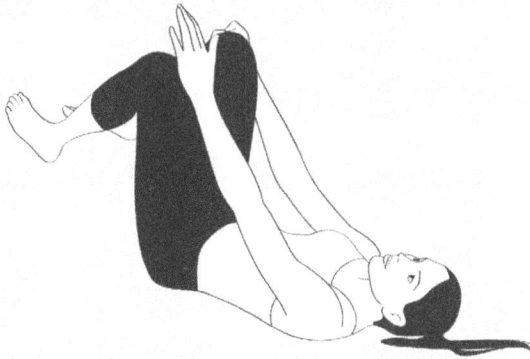

These instructions are assuming the SI joint pain is on your left side. If not, perform this technique on the right side.

Lie on the floor (not a bed) and bring your knees up.

Place one hand above the knee on your thigh and the other on your opposite leg below the knee.

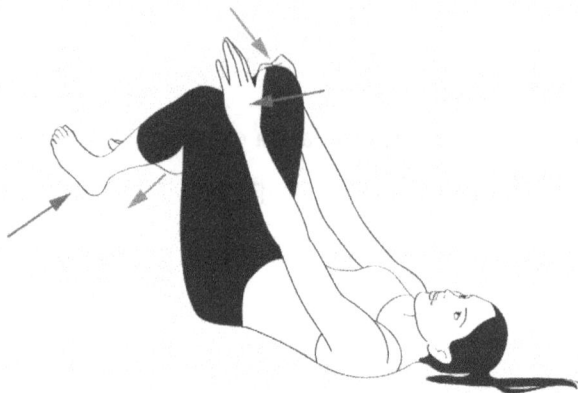

Press your legs against your hands with the added resistance.

Hold for 3 to 5 seconds and then release.

Repeat two to three times.

Technique #2

Static Back Knee Squeeze

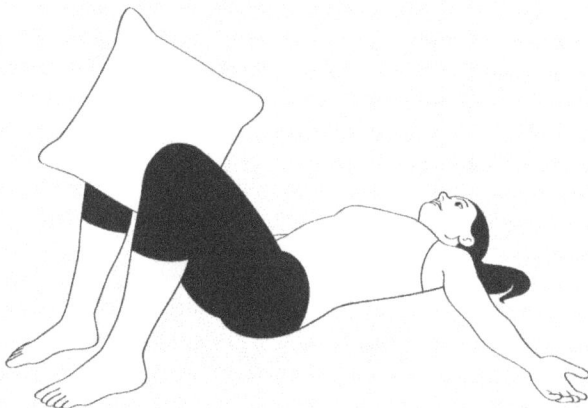

Lie with knees bent at a 90-degree angle. Place a thick pillow between your knees, and then, with your inner thigh muscles, gently squeeze the pillow for 15 seconds. Do three sets.

Helpful Tip: Try not to contract your stomach/abdominal muscles while squeezing.

REVERSE SCIATICA EXERCISE ROUTINE

Many of my massage clients come in for a treatment, hoping that my massage techniques will help loosen the muscles around the lower back and hip, taking the pressure off their sciatic nerve.

In some cases, my deep tissue massage can make a significant difference, but I always recommend weekly sessions for my clients to see a change.

To really get a lasting change, doing your own self-care routine will give you the real answer to how to relieve your sciatica.

For the best results, do the following 10 exercises every day until you feel a decrease in the sciatica pain.

1. Knees to Chest Stretch

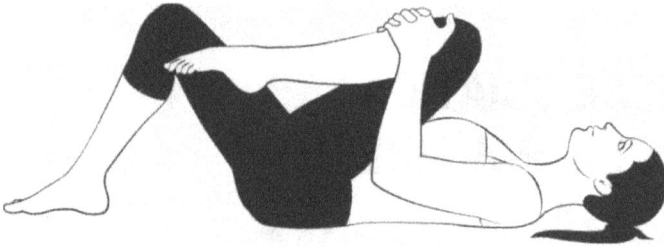

Lie on your back, with your knees bent. Grasp your left knee and pull it to your chest.

Hold for 20 to 30 seconds.

With your abdominals contracted, try to straighten your right leg. If you experience any discomfort in your back, leave your right leg bent.

Repeat this move with the other leg.

2. Hamstring Stretch with Yoga Strap (Contract-Relax)

When your hamstrings are tight, they pull your pelvis backward, thus affecting your lumbar spine or lower back.

Tight hamstrings pull on their attachment points, known as the ischial tuberosity. The ischial tuberosity is also known as the sitz bone, or as a pair, the sitting bones.

So, what happens when the pelvis tilts back and what's this mean for your hamstrings?

If the hamstrings are tight, the lumbar vertebrae inevitably become flexed forward. This can put unwanted strain on the lumbar spine and lead to bulging or herniated discs.

Contrarily, when the hamstrings are limber, the pelvis is able to freely tilt forward, so you bend from the hip joint and not the lumbar spine.

The importance of stretching your hamstrings shouldn't be ignored if you truly want to free yourself of low back pain or proactively prevent a future back spasm or hamstring pull.

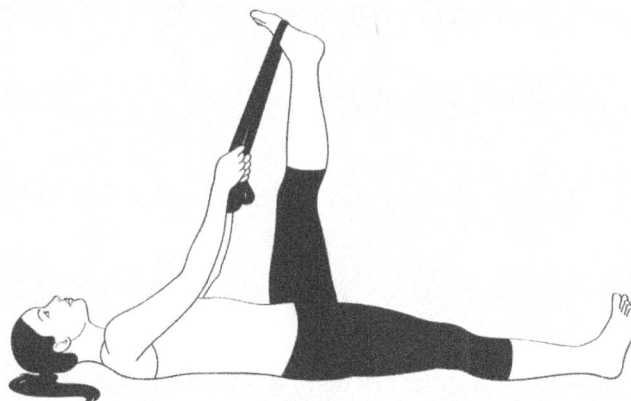

Using a yoga strap or stretch strap has been shown to be extremely effective at increasing the hamstring's flexibility and restoring range of motion.

To perform a proprioceptive neuromuscular facilitation (PNF) hamstring stretch (contract-relax antagonist-contract) using a strap, lie on your back and loop the strap around the ball of your foot, holding the ends of the strap with both hands.

Try to keep your chin down and your shoulders back. Exhale, while pushing your heel toward the ceiling. Hold this stretch for 20 to 30 seconds. Keeping your knee straight, push down with your heel into the strap toward the floor for 3 to 5 seconds. Then try to straighten your knee and actively push your foot toward the ceiling, contracting your quadriceps. Hold this for 3 to 5 seconds.

Relax and then hold this stretch for 20 to 30 seconds.

Repeat on the other leg.

3. Piriformis Stretch

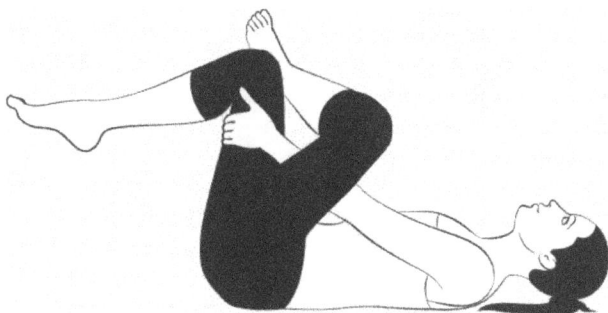

To stretch the piriformis, start by lying faceup on the floor, with your knees bent. Place your left foot on your right knee, and with both hands reach through and grab underneath your right knee.

Hold for 20 to 30 seconds.

4. Seated Hip Stretch

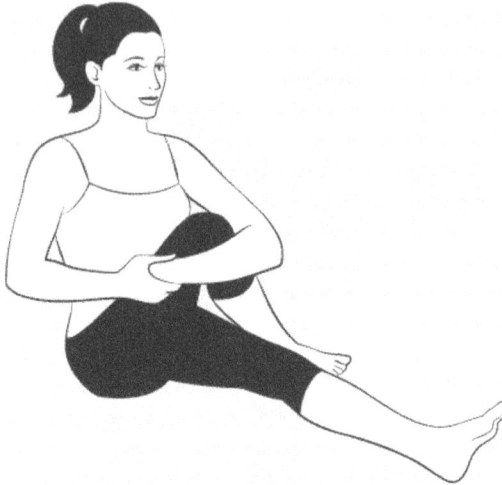

While in a sitting position, cross your right leg over your straightened left leg. Hug your right knee with your left arm, making sure to keep your back straight.

Hold this stretch for 30 to 60 seconds.

Repeat on the opposite side.

5. Pigeon Pose

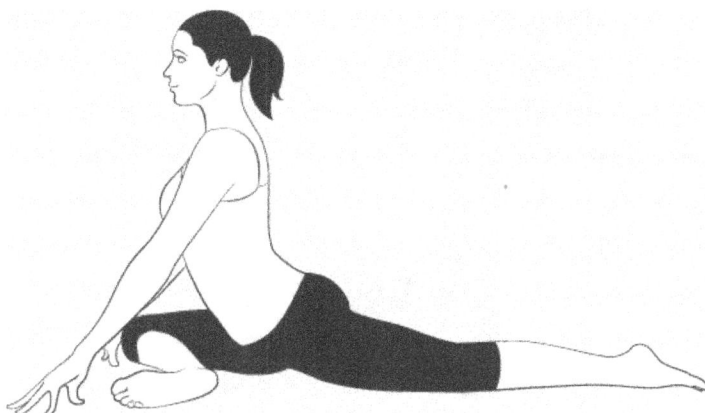

Start on your hands and knees, an all-fours position, with your hands slightly in front of your shoulders.

Draw your right knee forward and turn it out to the right, so your right leg is bent and your left leg is extended straight behind you.

Slowly lower both legs.

Hold the position for 5 to 10 breaths, and then switch to the other side.

If you find this Pigeon Pose stretch too intense or difficult, try a variation.

6. Fully Extended Press Up

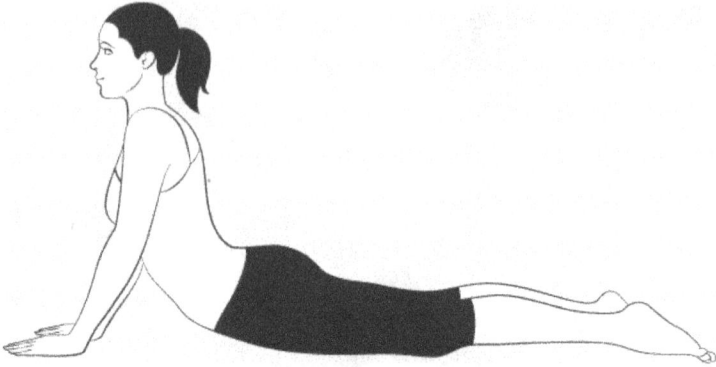

Press your palms into the floor and lift your upper body, keeping hips and pelvis rooted to the floor. Extend through the spine from the tailbone to the neck, allowing your back to arch.

Hold for 2 seconds, then slowly return to the start position for one repetition.

Do 10 repetitions.

7. Locust Pose

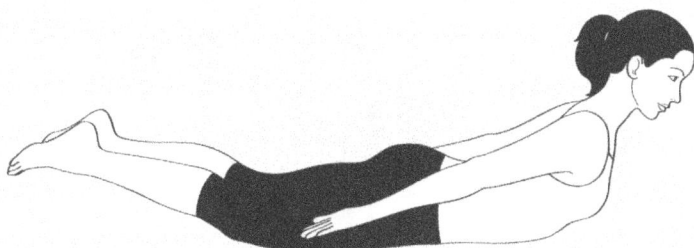

Lie on your stomach on the floor with your arms at your side. Lift your head and chest off the floor, tightly hold your glutes (buttock muscles), and squeeze your shoulder blades together.

Hold briefly and return to the start position.

Hold the Locust Pose for 15 to 20 seconds. Slowly release to the floor on an exhale.

Repeat two times.

8. Alternating Superman (or Superwoman) Exercise

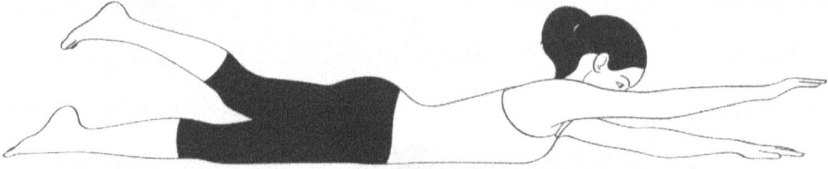

This exercise strengthens the erector spinae back muscles.

Lie face down on the floor on your stomach with arms and legs extended and your neck in a neutral position.

Lift opposite arm and leg for 3 to 5 seconds.

Repeat 10 to 20 times.

Repeat with the opposite arm and leg.

9. Donkey Kicks

Get down in the all-fours position.

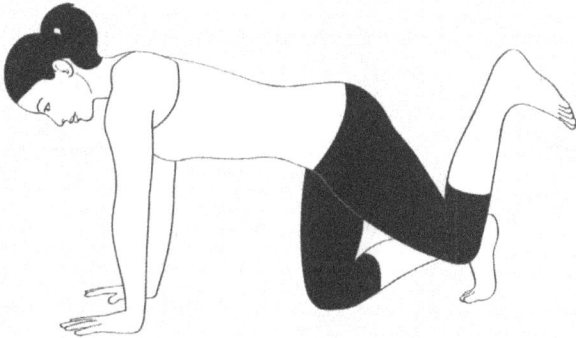

Kick your left leg straight back, while using your glute to raise your foot toward the ceiling.

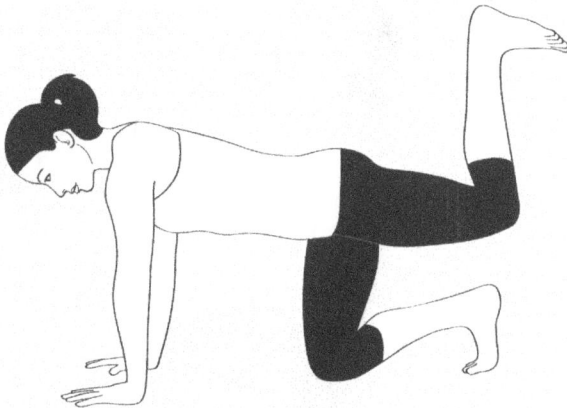

Hold for 1 second at the top, and slowly lower to starting position.

Do 15 to 20 repetitions on each leg.

See https://www.healthline.com/health/fitness-exercise/donkey-kick#2

10. Hip Flexor Stretch (with Arm Raised over Head)

Due to the predominant, sedentary culture we live in, most people's psoas muscle is chronically tight, pulling on the muscle attachments of the lower back. This can cause an imbalance in the pelvis that can ultimately lead to severe back pain or even a herniated disc.

Luckily, by doing this hip flexor stretch, it can help to reverse this phenomenon.

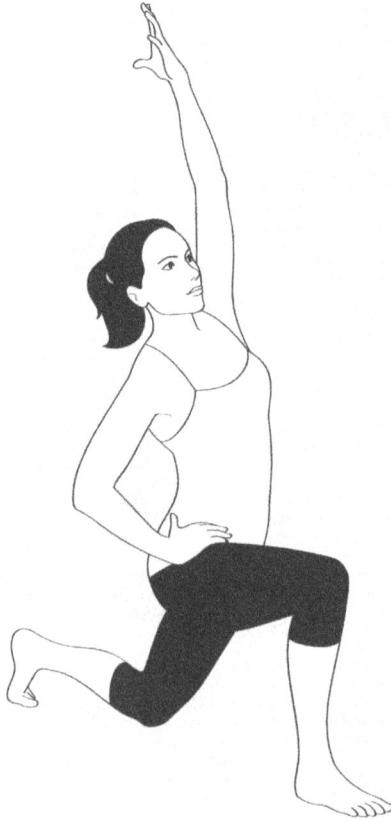

First, kneel on your right knee, with toes down, and place your left foot flat on the floor in front of you.

Place both hands on your left thigh and press your hips forward until you feel a good stretch in the hip flexors.

Reach your hands over your head and arch your body back.

Contract your abdominals and slightly tilt your pelvis back while keeping your chin parallel to the floor. Hold this pose for 30 seconds, and then switch sides. Stretch your nondominant side first.

TRIGGER-POINT SELF-MASSAGE TO RELIEVE SCIATICA

You can try trigger-point therapy using a tennis ball (or a lacrosse ball). Find a painful spot in the glutes, place the ball at that location, and then relax your body into the ball.

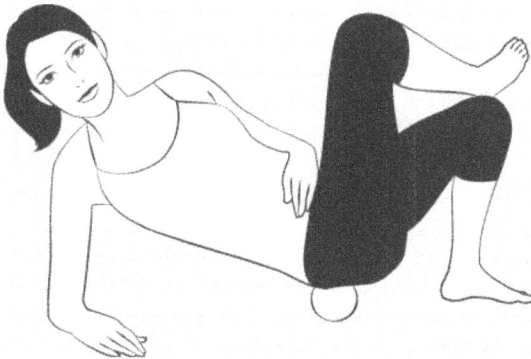

Focus on targeting the area closest to the sacrum and along the outside of the hip. If your leg starts to go numb, back off, as this indicates that you're irritating the sciatic nerve.

Once you find the painful spot, place the ball at that location, and then relax your body into the ball.

Hold this position for 20 to 30 seconds.

THIS ONE MOVE FIXES OVERLY TIGHT HIP FLEXORS

A common complaint I get from a number of my clients is, "Morgan, my hips are so tight."

And my normal response is, "Here, try this hip flexor stretch." And that's when I recommend the classic kneeling hip flexor stretch. (See images and instructions for the Hip Flexor Stretch on page 11 or page 84.)

Question

Why do your hips get so tight?

Short Answer

From all that sitting you've been doing.

If you spend hours on end in a seated position, you're constantly contracting your hip flexors, which causes them to get shorter.

The average person spends at least a third of the day sitting. Now, think about all that time their hip flexor muscles stay shortened.

Way too much, right?

Their hip flexors inevitably become tighter and tighter until the concept of standing up straight is impossible

So, unless you want to look like that, I want you to practice this one move that will fix your over-tight hip flexors.

Supine Groin Stretch

This is a great exercise if you have been struggling to stretch your hip flexors and also suffering from chronic low back pain.

The supine groin stretch is a perfect choice if your pain seems to come on suddenly and increases when you lift your thigh toward your chest.

I know 5 minutes might be a lot, but, nonetheless, it will help you decompress after a long day.

If you're short on time, then do a 30-second kneeling hip flexor stretch.

How to Do the Supine Groin Stretch

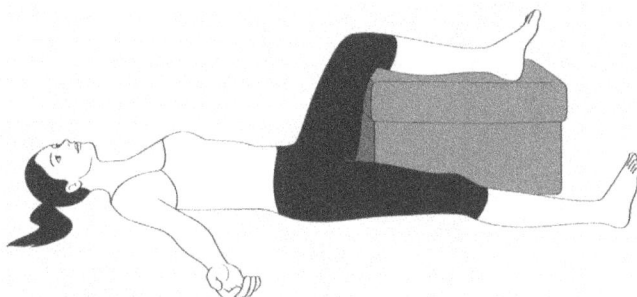

Start by lying flat on the floor with your arms at 45 degree angles from your body, palms up.

If your right hip flexor is the tight one, then place your left knee on a chair or ottoman

Make sure your hip and knee are a 90-degree angle.

Now, relax your foot against an object, like a thick cushion or a small weight.

The point is to keep the toe pointing up, so it doesn't twist, making the stretch less effective.

Next, do a quick quad test, where you contract the thigh of the leg that is on the floor for a second, then relax. You will likely feel this close to your knee.

Now, lie there and relax for the next 5 minutes. When the 5 minutes is up, do the quad test again.

Repeat these steps until you feel the contraction closer to the middle or even the top of the thigh.

Eventually, you should feel your quad contract higher up your thigh, in the hip pocket region.

FOUR RESISTANCE BAND STRENGTHENING EXERCISES FOR SCIATICA RELIEF

What You Need

One long elastic band and one resistance band loop (red/medium or green/advanced)—see Resources for a link to purchase bands.

1. Bridge with Resistance Band

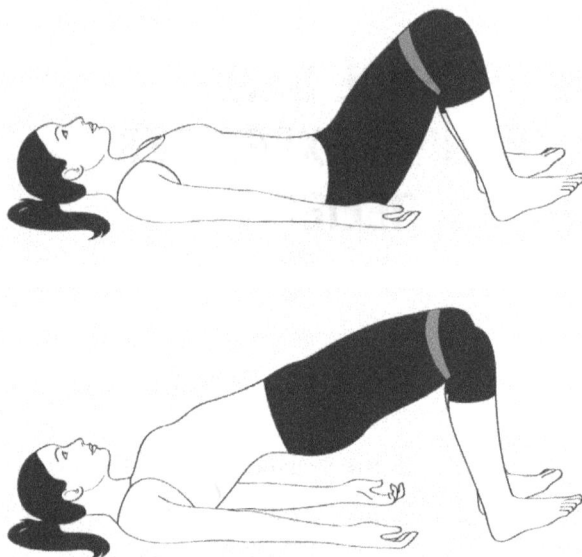

Loop the band tightly around your knees. Separate your knees against the resistance from the band, squeeze your butt together, and perform a bridge by lifting your buttocks off the floor.

Slowly return to start position.

Repeat 15 to 20 times.

2. The Clam Shell—Resisted Hip Abduction (Lying Down)

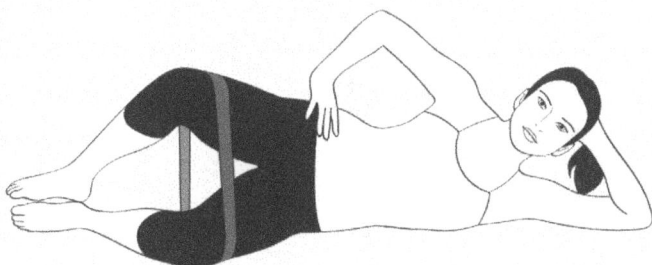

The Clam Shell strengthens hip abductors, because you are lifting them against gravity.

Lie on your side, with your knees pointed forward and bent at a 90-degree angle. Place the resistance band around your knees.

Lift your top knee upward about 8 to 12 inches, making sure your upper foot stays in place against your lower foot.

Lower your upper knee to the bottom knee. This completes one repetition.

Repeat 15 to 20 times.

Then switch sides.

3. Resisted Hip Abduction (Standing)

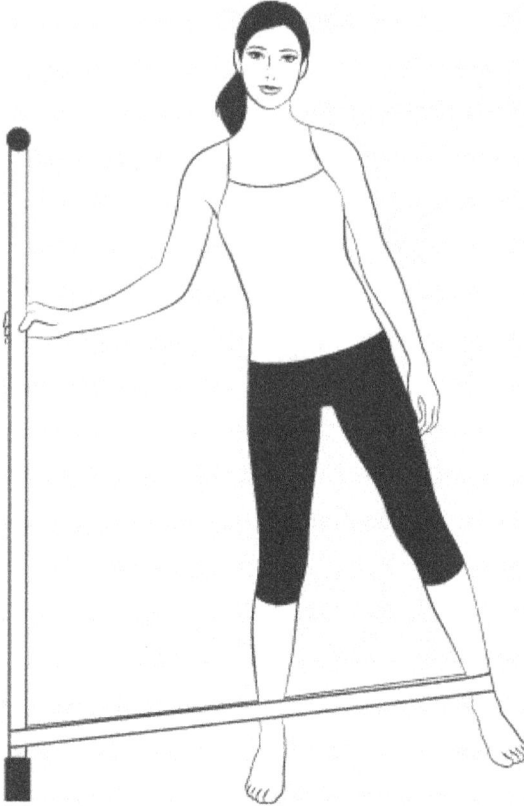

TheraBand hip abductions strengthen the outside of the hip muscles, which help externally rotate and lift your legs to the side.

Start by looping one end of the resistance band around a sturdy object and the other end around your ankle. Stand tall with the looped ankle farthest from the opposite end of the band while holding the sturdy object with your inside arm.

Lift your outer leg straight out to side as far as possible.

Pause, then return your leg to the starting position.

Do 15 to 20 repetitions on each side.

See https://www.muscleandfitness.com/workouts/abs-and-core-exercises/videos/standing-resistance-band-hip-abduction

4. Resisted Hip Extension (Standing)

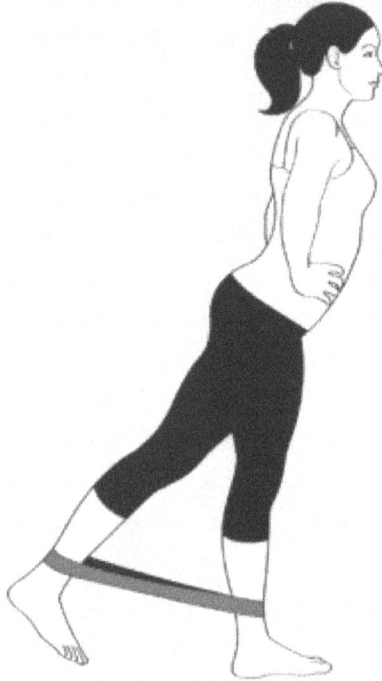

This hip extension exercise strengthens the large buttock muscles and also the hamstrings on the back of the thigh.

Stand with the band around one ankle and attached to a fixed point in front. Use something to hold onto (like a wall), if you need to.

Keeping the leg straight, extend the hip as far as comfortable and return to the start position.

Keep the hips facing forward and perform the exercise in a slow and controlled manner. You should feel it working the buttock muscles.

Repeat 15 to 20 times.

Switch to the other leg, and then do another 15 to 20 repetitions.

FIX YOUR POSTURE, FIX YOUR KNEES

Next to back and neck pain, knee pain is the most common site of pain and disability in the legs.

When knee problems occur, and a person loses their full range of pain-free movement, functional strength and their quality of life is dramatically affected.

Night after night of disturbed sleep drives many knee pain sufferers to take medication, stop work, and let go of activities that give them joy.

Abandoning active lifestyles due to knee pain ultimately leads to reduced fitness and weight gain, which will further impact their knee problems.

The supportive structures of the knee are susceptible to injury, mainly when a person wrenches it while performing a forceful twisting motion.

Injuries can occur while slipping on a wet surface, playing a sport, or falling directly onto the knee, resulting in a potential ligament and meniscus tear.

Prolonged Standing

Specific injuries are not the only cause for knee pain. Postural neglect plays a significant role as one of the common causes of knee pain.

Prolonged standing positions limit the range of motion and can gradually make the knee joint weaker, making it lose its shock-absorbing capacity.

Suddenly increasing the load on the knee, as in jumping or going into a deep squat, the knees can become overloaded, causing pain.

Prolonged Sitting

A 2016 study publishing in the *Journal of Orthopaedic & Sports Physical Therapy* found that the average adult spends 14 hours a day sitting. Inactivity and low fitness levels are several factors that lead to the development of knee pain.

Prolonged sitting postures with the knees bent for an extended period will eventually overstretch and overload the structures in and around the knee.

Being stationary for extended periods can lead to stiffness and pain when rising from a seated position, and if the bent posture continues, the knee might even become painful while sitting.

See https://www.jospt.org/doi/full/10.2519/jospt.2016.6470

Poor Sleeping Posture

The structures in and around the knee can also become overstretched and overloaded while lying in a sleeping position, because the knee is bent for an extended period.

Helpful Tip: Placing a pillow between the knees instead of letting the knees press together is a simple solution.

If this doesn't do the trick, then lying supine with a pillow under your knees can help ease the pain.

Being Overweight

Being overweight has been linked to the onset of knee pain by the American Academy of Orthopaedic Surgeons (AAOS).

Studies say that having a body mass index (BMI) over 25 points is associated with an increased risk of knee pain accompanied by loss of function.

If a person has a BMI higher than 25, the AAOS suggests a 5 percent weight loss, and this can help decrease knee pain.

What We Can Learn about Knee Pain by Watching Children Move

Watch a four-year-old child, and you will instantly notice how active they are and how they are naturally inclined to be always moving.

When recess rolls around, what do they do? Sit on their bums and veg out?

Nope!

They run around like bolts of lightning and hop, skip, and jump.

This is a learning opportunity for knee pain sufferers. Instead of resting the knee by doing less, activity is essential to reversing the debilitating effects of knee pain.

EIGHT DEAD SIMPLE EXERCISES FOR KNEE PAIN RELIEF

The following exercises are taken from *Treat Your Own Knee* by Robin McKenzie, a New Zealand-born physiotherapist whose McKenzie Method is currently the most studied diagnostic treatment system for back pain.

This knee pain exercise program will allow you to treat your knee pain and regain pain-free movement.

Important Note: For optimal knee pain relief, do the following stretches 10 times every two hours throughout the day until you go to bed.

Exercise 1: Active Knee Extension in Sitting

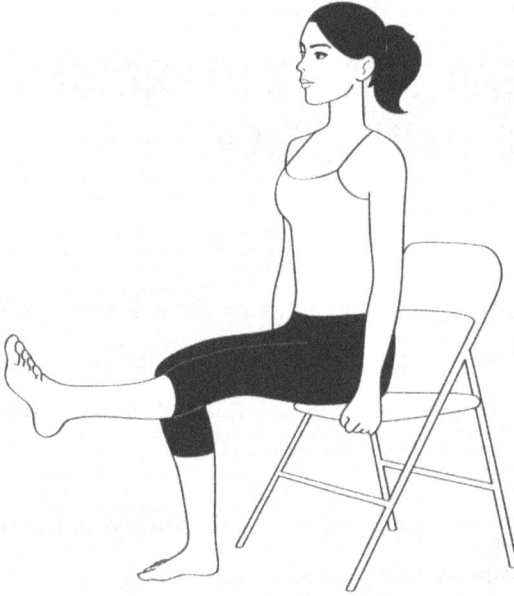

Start by sitting upright in a chair with your feet flat on the floor.

Slowly lift the foot of your painful knee and straighten your leg until you feel your quadriceps (thighs) contract.

Hold for 2 seconds and then return your foot to the starting position.

Repeat 10 times.

Exercise 2: Knee Extension in Sitting

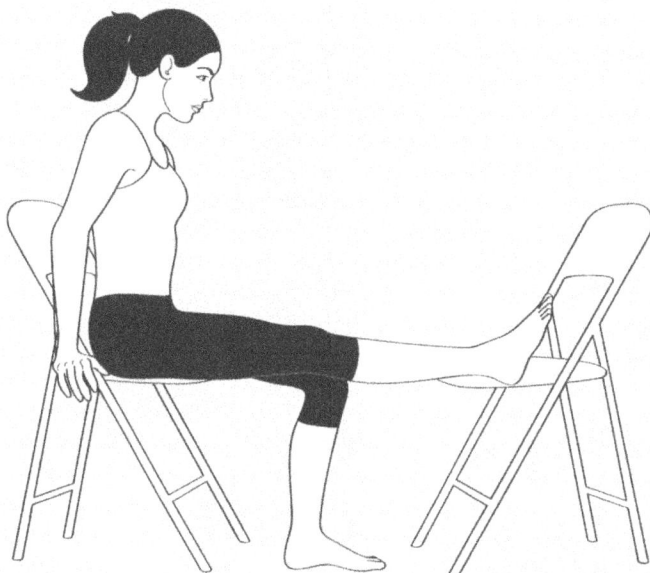

Sit in a chair and place the heel of the painful knee on a chair or stool of similar height with your knee slightly bent and toes pointing up.

With a relaxed knee, slowly straighten your leg.

Hold for 2 seconds and then return your knee to the starting position.

Repeat 10 times.

Now, reach forward with both hands and place them just above your knee.

Slowly push down and straighten your knee with your hands until you feel a slight stretch behind the knee.

97

Hold for 2 seconds and return to the starting position.

Repeat 10 times.

Helpful Tip: Remember to move just into the pain and then release the pressure.

Exercise 3: Knee Extension in Standing

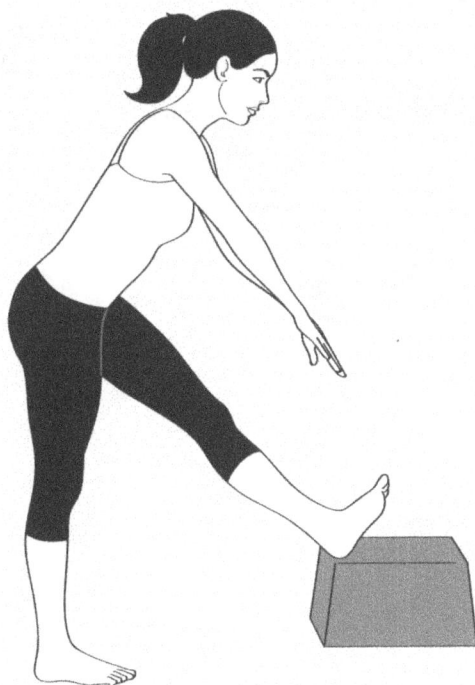

Stand upright and place the heel of your painful knee on a low stepstool or on the floor.

Slowly reach forward with both hands, placing them just above your knee.

Slowly push down and straighten your knee with your hands until you feel a good knee stretch.

Hold for 2 seconds and return to the starting position.

Repeat 10 times.

If your pain is on the inside of the knee, rotate your foot outward while doing this knee extension exercise.

If your pain is on the outside of the knee, turn your foot inward while doing this knee extension exercise.

Exercise 4: Knee Flexion in Sitting

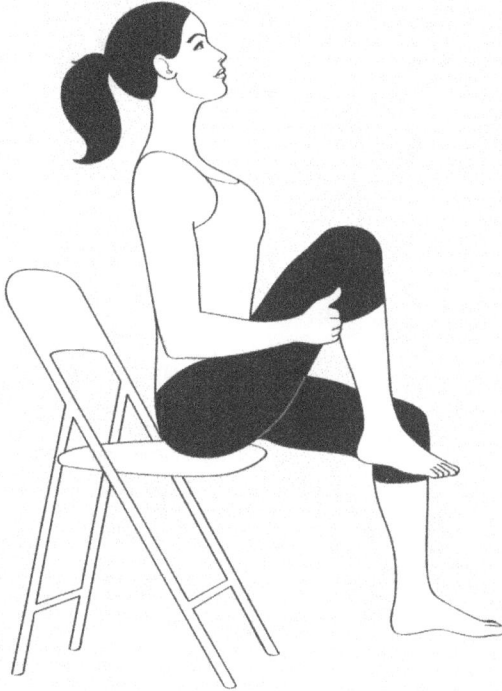

Begin by sitting in an upright position.

Slowly bend your knee. With both hands, pull your leg toward your chest.

Pull your heel toward your buttocks and hold for 2 seconds.

Then return your knee to the starting position.

Repeat 10 times.

Helpful Tip: You can place a rolled-up towel behind your knee for added comfort and to create a little bit of space in the knee joint.

Exercise 5: Standing Quadriceps Stretch

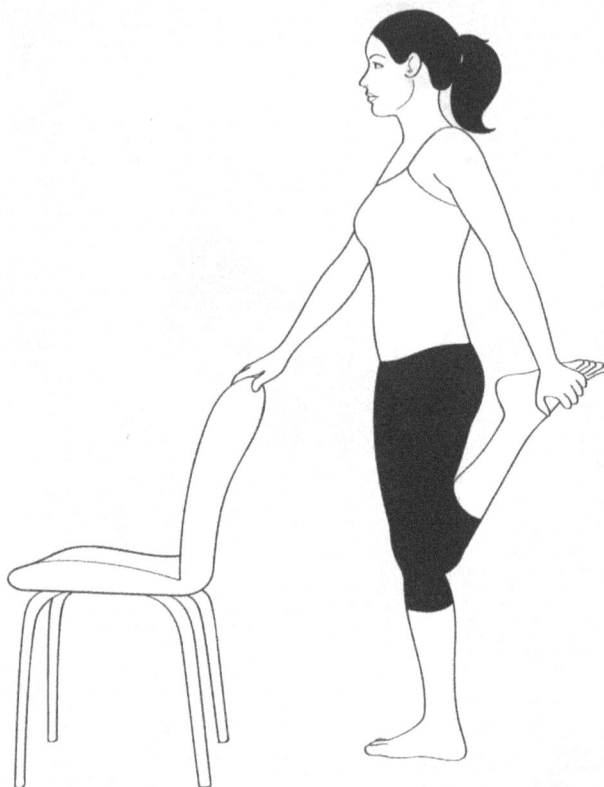

Stand upright and place the heel of your painful knee on a chair or a stool. If needed, hold on to the chair for balance.

Slowly lean forward and push your buttock toward your heel until you feel a good knee stretch.

Hold for 2 seconds.

Repeat 10 times.

Helpful Tip: If this exercise is uncomfortable, try placing a rolled-up hand towel behind the knee, and this should relieve the discomfort.

Exercise 6: Knee Flexion in Kneeling

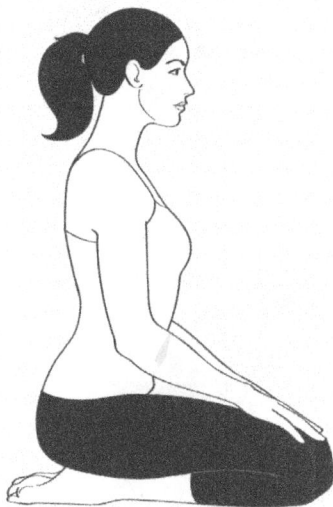

Start kneeling on all fours, with a cushion underneath your knees for support.

Slowly kneel back onto your heels with your hands on the floor in front of you. You should feel a firm stretch in your knees.

Hold this position for 2 seconds

Repeat 6 to 10 times.

Now, do the stretch again, but this time lift your hands off the floor and sit on your heels.

Hold for 2 seconds, then return to the starting position.

Repeat 10 times.

Exercise 7: Chair Squats

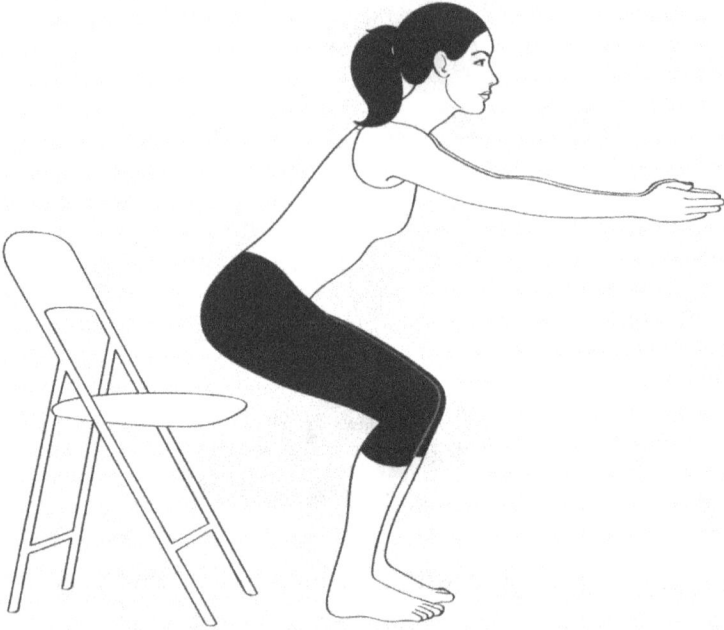

Stand upright with feet shoulder-width apart and a chair behind you.

Slowly sit back until you feel a firm tension in the muscles around your knee.

Remember to keep your knees pointing forward as you lower your hips toward the chair, but don't sit.

Repeat 10–15 times, twice a day.

Exercise 8: Single-Leg Squats

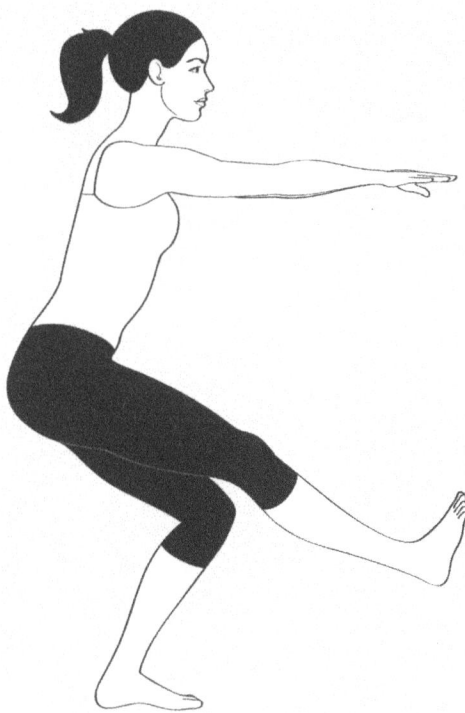

Stand upright on the leg with the knee pain.

Do 5 or 10 single-leg squats, being sure to keep your torso upright and your knee about level with your toes.

Great job! Now you're on the road to recovery to experiencing knee pain relief.

CONCLUSION

Taking ownership of your pain is essential to living a pain-free life. I hope that the various ways illustrated in this book have empowered you to take action so you can feel like yourself again.

As the old saying goes, "motion is lotion for the joints." What that means is that the older you get, the less lubrication (or synovial fluid) you produce for your joints. And the little fluid you do produce isn't absorbed as well by the joints, so the more active you are, the better you'll feel overall.

Watch some young children, and you'll instantly notice how active they are and how they're naturally inclined to be constantly moving. When recess rolls around, what do they do? Sit on their bums and veg out? Nope! They run around like bolts of lightning and hop, skip, and jump.

This is a learning opportunity for back, hip, and knee pain sufferers. Instead of resting and doing less, activity is essential to reversing the debilitating effects of poor posture.

I wish you well on your journey to health and well-being!

REFERENCES

Got Back Pain? Now What?

Bichell, Rae Ellen. (2016). "Forget the Gizmos: Exercise Works Best for Lower-Back Pain."
See
http://www.npr.org/sections/healthshots/2016/01/11/462366361/forget-the-gizmos-exercise-works-best-for-lower-back-pain.

Cole, Andrew J. (2000). "The Myths and Reality of Back Pain and Back Problems."
See http://www.spine-health.com/conditions/lower-back-pain/myths-and-reality-back-pain-and-back-problems.

Deardorff, William W. (2017). "Types of Back Pain: Acute Pain, Chronic Pain, and Neuropathic Pain."
See http://www.spine-health.com/conditions/chronic-pain/types-back-pain-acute-pain-chronic-pain-and-neuropathic-pain.

"Handout on Health: Back Pain." (2013). National Institutes of Health (NIH): National Institute of Arthritis and Musculoskeletal and Skin Diseases.
See http://www.niams.nih.gov/Health_Info/Back_Pain/default.asp.

Hoy, D., Bain, C., Williams, G., March, L., Brooks, P., Blyth, F. Woolf, A., Vos, T., Buchbinder, R. (2012). "A Systemic Review of the Global Prevalence of Low Back Pain." *Arthritis & Rheumatology* 64, no. 6, 2028–2037. doi: 10.1002/art.34347.

Institute of Medicine of the National Academies (2011). *Relieving Pain in America, A Blueprint for Transforming Prevention, Care, Education, and Research.* Washington, DC: The National Academies Press.

"Low Back Pain Fact Sheet." (2003). National Institutes of Health (NIH): National Institute of Neurological Disorders and Stroke. See http://www.ninds.nih.gov/disorders/backpain/detail_backpain.htm.

"Low Back Pain Fact Sheet." (2014). National Institute of Neurological Disorders and Stroke.
See
http://www.ninds.nih.gov/disorders/backpain/detail_backpain.htm.

Malmivaara, A., Häkkinen, U., Aro, T., Heinrichs, M-L., Koskenniemi, L., Kuosma, E., Lappi, S., Paloheimo, R., Servo, C., Vaaranen, V., and Hernberg, S., (1995). "The Treatment of Acute Low Back Pain—Bed Rest, Exercises, or Ordinary Activity?" *The New England Journal of Medicine* 332, 351–355.

Steffens, D., Maher, C.G., Pereira, L.S.M. (2016). "Prevention of Low Back Pain: A Systematic Review and Meta-analysis." *JAMA Intern Med* 176, no. 2,199–208. doi: 10.1001/jamainternmed.2015.7431

Four Most Common Causes of Back Pain

McKenzie, Robin A. (2011). *Treat Your Own Back*. Orthopedic Physical Therapy Products.

Twenty-One Day, Low Back Pain, Relief Program

"Adductor Assisted Back Extension." (2014). See https://www.youtube.com/watch?v=mZr5ywYLSwQ.

Ameel. (2012).

Ferris, Tim. (2010). *The Four-Hour Body: An Uncommon Guide to Rapid Fat-Loss, Incredible Sex, and Becoming Superhuman*. Harmony, 352.

Goodman, Eric. (2011). *Foundation: Redefine Your Core, Conquer Back Pain, and Move with Confidence*. Rodale Books, 96–97.

"Hamstring Stretches." See http://www.stretching-exercises-guide.com/hamstring-stretches.html.

Koch, Nathan. (2014). "New Runner: Dynamic Stretching vs. Static Stretching." See http://running.competitor.com/2014/07/injury-prevention/dynamic-stretching-vs-static-stretching_54248#uHp6YUjcUOp00fxy.99.

"Lumbar/Core Strength and Stability Exercises." See https://uhs.princeton.edu/sites/uhs/files/documents/Lumbar.pdf.

Samartzis, D., Karppinen, J., Chan, D., Luk, K.D.K., and Cheung, K.M.C. (2012). "The Association of Lumbar Intervertebral Disc Degeneration on Magnetic Resonance Imaging with Body Mass Index in Overweight and Obese Adults: A Population-Based Study." *Arthritis & Rheumatology* 64, no. 5, 1488–1496. doi: 10.1002/art.33462.

Shiri, R., Karppinen, J., Leino-Arjas, P., Solovieva, S., and Viikari-Juntura, E. (2010). "The Association between Obesity and Low Back Pain: A Meta-Analysis." *American Journal of Epidemiology* 171, no. 2, 135–154. doi: 10.1093/aje/kwp356.

Shiri, R., Solovieva, S., Husgafvel-Pursiainen, K., Taimela, S., Saarikoski, L.A., Huupponen, R., Viikari, J., Raitakari, O.T., and Viikari-Juntura, E. (2008). "The Association between Obesity and the Prevalence of Low Back Pain in Young Adults: The Cardiovascular Risk in Young Finns Study." *American Journal of Epidemiology* 167, no. 9, 1110–1119. doi: 10.1093/aje/kwn007.

"Weak Posterior Kinetic Chain: Cause of Lower Back Pain."
See http://backpainsolutionsonline.com/announcements-and-releases/backpain/lower-back-pain-causes/weak-posterior-kinetic-chain-cause-of-lower-back-pain.

Westbrock, H. (2015). "The Best Stretch for Your Hip Flexors—The 'Couch Stretch.'"
See https://premiersportsandspine.com/2015/06/the-best-stretch-for-your-hip-flexors-the-couch-stretch/.

Hamstring Stretch with Yoga Strap (Contract-Relax)

Stretching Exercises Guide. "Hamstring Stretches."
See http://www.stretching-exercises-guide.com/hamstring-stretches.html

Locust Pose

Marla. (2009). "Learn to Backbend Better: Locust Pose."
See http://www.yogajournal.com/article/beginners/locust-pose/

Resistance Bands

Page, Phil. (2011). "Thera-Band Exercises Effective for Piriformis Syndrome."
See http://www.hygenicblog.com/2011/01/12/thera-band-exercises-effective-for-piriformis-syndrome/

Donkey Kicks

"Donkey Kicks with Flat Bands."
See https://bodylastics.com/exercises/donkey-kicks-with-flat-resistance-bands/

Six Foam Rolling Moves to Conquer Back Pain

"How to Foam Roll Your Hamstrings." (2013).
See https://www.youtube.com/watch?v=fMfe6DnlGvA.

Macdonald, G.Z., Button, D.C., Drinkwater, E.J., and Behm, D.G. (2014). "Foam Rolling as a Recovery Tool after an Intense Bout of Physical Activity." *Medicine & Science in Sports & Exercise* 46, no. 1, 131–142. doi: 10.1249/MSS.0b013e3182a123db.

Starrett, Kelly. (2015). *Becoming a Supple Leopard: The Ultimate Guide to Resolving Pain, Preventing Injury, and Optimizing Athletic Performance*. Victory Belt Publishing.

The Six-Minute Emergency Back Pain Treatment

Fanslau, Jill. (2016). "The Fit Man's Back-Saving Workout." See http://www.menshealth.com/fitness/exercises-to-prevent-back-pain?_ga=1.156404476.652772678.1492037609.

McKenzie, Robin A. (2011). *Treat Your Own Back*. Orthopedic Physical Therapy Products.

Fix Your Posture, Fix Your Knee

McKenzie, Robin. (2012). *Treat Your Own Knee*. Orthopedic Physical Therapy Products.

Eight Dead Simple Exercises for Knee Pain Relief

McKenzie, Robin. (2012). *Treat Your Own Knee*. Orthopedic Physical Therapy Products.

Miller, Jill. "The Stretch That Will Make Your Knees Feel 10 Years Younger." (2014).
See https://www.youtube.com/watch?v=reanPMXGqcA.

RESOURCES

To fully take advantage of these back pain relief exercises, I highly recommend you get the following supplies.

Foam roller for self-massage
http://amzn.to/2ntTByb

Stretch strap
http://amzn.to/2nGFwwF

Beginner set of resistance bands
http://amzn.to/2ncfAw9

TheraBand loops
http://amzn.to/2nGs8Zt

Yoga mat
http://amzn.to/2n1xOQF

Memory foam mattress for quality sleep
http://amzn.to/2pkOsbi

ABOUT THE AUTHOR

Since becoming a professional massage therapist in 2000, Morgan Sutherland has consistently helped thousands of clients manage their back pain with a combination of deep tissue work, cupping, and stretching. In 2002, he began a career-long tradition of continuing study by being trained in Tuina—the art of Chinese massage—at the world-famous Olympic Training Center in Beijing, China.

As an orthopedic massage therapist, Morgan specializes in treating chronic pain and sports injuries and helping restore proper range of motion. In 2006, Morgan became certified as a medical massage practitioner, giving him the knowledge and ability to work with physicians in a complementary healthcare partnership.

When he's not helping clients manage their back pain, he's writing blog posts about pain relief and self-care, in addition to teaching live and virtual workshops on how to incorporate massage cupping into a bodywork practice. Morgan has received the Angie's List Super Service Award for 2011, 2012, 2013, 2014, and 2015.

Morgan welcomes all comments about your real-life experiences implementing the stretches and exercises contained within this book. Thank you for reading.

Website: www.morganmassage.com
Email: morgan@morganmassage.com

OTHER BOOKS BY MORGAN SUTHERLAND, L.M.T.

The Essential Lower Back Pain Exercises Guide: Treat Low Back Pain at Home in Just Twenty-One Days

THIS Is How to Fix Bad Posture: The Best Exercises for Bad Posture That Your Mother Never Taught You

21 Yoga Exercises for Lower Back Pain: Stretching Lower Back Pain Away with Yoga

Reverse Bad Posture Exercises: Fix Neck, Back, and Shoulder Pain in Just 15 Minutes Per Day, Reverse Your Pain Book 1

Best Treatment for Sciatica Pain: Relieve Sciatica Symptoms, Piriformis Muscle Pain, and SI Joint Pain in Just 15 Minutes Per Day

Resistance Band Workouts for Bad Posture and Back Pain: An Illustrated Resistance Band Exercise Book for Better Posture and Back Pain Relief

DIY Low Back Pain Relief: 9 Ways to Fix Low Back Pain So You Can Feel Like Yourself Again

www.ingramcontent.com/pod-product-compliance
Lightning Source LLC
Chambersburg PA
CBHW060243030426
42335CB00014B/1582